Tumors of the Ear and Lateral Skull Base, Part 1

Editors

GEORGE B. WANNA
MATTHEW LUKE CARLSON

OTOLARYNGOLOGIC CLINICS OF NORTH AMERICA

www.oto.theclinics.com

April 2015 • Volume 48 • Number 2

ELSEVIER

1600 John F. Kennedy Boulevard • Suite 1800 • Philadelphia, Pennsylvania, 19103-2899

http://www.oto.theclinics.com

OTOLARYNGOLOGIC CLINICS OF NORTH AMERICA Volume 48, Number 2
April 2015 ISSN 0030-6665, ISBN-13: 978-0-323-35980-1

Editor: Joanne Husovski
Developmental Editor: Susan Showalter

Otolaryngologic Clinics of North America (ISSN 0030-6665) is published bimonthly by Elsevier, Inc., 360 Park Avenue South, New York, NY 10010-1710. Months of issue are February, April, June, August, October, and December. Business and Editorial Offices: 1600 John F. Kennedy Blvd., Suite 1800, Philadelphia, PA 19103-2899. Customer Service Office: 6277 Sea Harbor Drive, Orlando, FL 32887-4800. Periodicals postage paid at New York, NY and additional mailing offices. Subscription prices is $365.00 per year (US individuals), $692.00 per year (US institutions), $175.00 per year (US student/resident), $485.00 per year (Canadian individuals), $876.00 per year (Canadian institutions), $540.00 per year (international individuals), $876.00 per year (international institutions), $270.00 per year (international & Canadian student/resident). Foreign air speed delivery is included in all *Clinics'* subscription prices. All prices are subject to change without notice. **POSTMASTER:** Send address changes to *Otolaryngologic Clinics of North America*, Elsevier Health Sciences Division, Subscription Customer Service, 3251 Riverport Lane, Maryland Heights, MO 63043. **Telephone: 1-800-654-2452 (U.S. and Canada); 314-447-8871 (outside U.S. and Canada). Fax: 314-447-8029. E-mail: journalscustomerservice-usa@elsevier.com (for print support); journalsonlinesupport-usa@elsevier.com (for online support).**

Reprints. For copies of 100 or more of articles in this publication, please contact the Commercial Reprints Department, Elsevier Inc., 360 Park Avenue South, New York, NY 10010-1710. Tel.: 212-633-3874; Fax: 212-633-3820; E-mail: reprints@elsevier.com.

Otolaryngologic Clinics of North America is also published in Spanish by McGraw-Hill Interamericana Editores S.A., P.O. Box 5-237, 06500 Mexico D.F., Mexico.

Otolaryngologic Clinics of North America is covered in *MEDLINE/PubMed (Index Medicus), Current Contents/Clinical Medicine, Excerpta Medica, BIOSIS, Science Citation Index,* and *ISI/BIOMED.*

PROGRAM OBJECTIVE

The goal of the *Otolaryngologic Clinics of North America* is to provide information on the latest trends in patient management, the newest advances; and provide a sound basis for choosing treatment options in the field of otolaryngology.

TARGET AUDIENCE

All practicing physicians and healthcare professionals who provide patient care to otolaryngologic patients.

LEARNING OBJECTIVES

Upon completion of this activity, participants will be able to:

1. Review innovations in tumor imaging.
2. Discuss the management of tumors of the ear and skull base.
3. Recognize and differentiate between the various types of tumors of ear and skull base.

ACCREDITATION

The Elsevier Office of Continuing Medical Education (EOCME) is accredited by the Accreditation Council for Continuing Medical Education (ACCME) to provide continuing medical education for physicians.

The EOCME designates this enduring material for a maximum of 15 *AMA PRA Category 1 Credit*(s)™. Physicians should claim only the credit commensurate with the extent of their participation in the activity.

All other health care professionals requesting continuing education credit for this enduring material will be issued a certificate of participation.

DISCLOSURE OF CONFLICTS OF INTEREST

The EOCME assesses conflict of interest with its instructors, faculty, planners, and other individuals who are in a position to control the content of CME activities. All relevant conflicts of interest that are identified are thoroughly vetted by EOCME for fair balance, scientific objectivity, and patient care recommendations. EOCME is committed to providing its learners with CME activities that promote improvements or quality in healthcare and not a specific proprietary business or a commercial interest.

The planning committee, staff, authors and editors listed below have identified no financial relationships or relationships to products or devices they or their spouse/life partner have with commercial interest related to the content of this CME activity:

Marc L. Bennett, MD; Jason A. Beyea, MD, PhD; Joseph T. Breen, MD; Matthew Luke Carlson, MD; C. Eduardo Corrales, MD; Nancy Fischbein, MD; Anjali Fortna; Michael B. Gluth, MD, FACS; Richard K. Gurgel, MD; David S. Haynes, MD, FACS; Kristen Helm; Brynne Hunter; Joanne Husovski; Robert K. Jackler, MD; Shira Koss, MD; Nauman F. Manzoor, MD; Cliff A. Megerian, MD, FACS; Aaron C. Moberly, MD; Stanley Pelosi, MD; Santha Priya; Maroun T. Semaan, MD, FACS; Susan Showalter; Alex D. Sweeney, MD; Andrew J. Thomas, MD; Jeffrey T. Vrabec, MD; George B. Wanna, MD, FACS; Cameron C. Wick, MD; Richard H. Wiggins, III, MD.

The planning committee, staff, authors and editors listed below have identified financial relationships or relationships to products or devices they or their spouse/life partner have with commercial interest related to the content of this CME activity:

Brandon Isaacson, MD, FACS: consultant/advisor for Advanced Bionics AG and Medtronic plc, employment affiliation at Stryker

UNAPPROVED/OFF-LABEL USE DISCLOSURE

The EOCME requires CME faculty to disclose to the participants:

1. When products or procedures being discussed are off-label, unlabelled, experimental, and/or investigational (not US Food and Drug Administration [FDA] approved); and
2. Any limitations on the information presented, such as data that are preliminary or that represent ongoing research, interim analyses, and/or unsupported opinions. Faculty may discuss information about pharmaceutical agents that is outside of FDA-approved labelling. This information is intended solely for CME and is not intended to promote off-label use of these medications. If you have any questions, contact the medical affairs department of the manufacturer for the most recent prescribing information.

TO ENROLL

To enroll in the *Otolaryngologic Clinics of North America* Continuing Medical Education program, call customer service at 1-800-654-2452 or sign up online at http://www.theclinics.com/home/cme. The CME program is available to subscribers for an additional annual fee of USD 260.

METHOD OF PARTICIPATION

In order to claim credit, participants must complete the following:

1. Complete enrolment as indicated above.
2. Read the activity.
3. Complete the CME Test and Evaluation. Participants must achieve a score of 70% on the test. All CME Tests and Evaluations must be completed online.

CME INQUIRIES/SPECIAL NEEDS

For all CME inquiries or special needs, please contact elsevierCME@elsevier.com.

Contributors

EDITOR

GEORGE B. WANNA, MD, FACS
Associate Professor, Department of Otolaryngology-Head and Neck Surgery, Division of Otology–Neurotology & Skull Base Surgery; Co-Director, Neurotology Fellowship Program; Vanderbilt University, Nashville, Tennessee

MATTHEW L. CARLSON, MD
Assistant Professor, Department of Otolaryngology-Head and Neck Surgery, Mayo Clinic School of Medicine, Rochester, Minnesota

AUTHORS

MARC L. BENNETT, MD
Department of Otolaryngology-Head and Neck Surgery, Vanderbilt University, Nashville, Tennessee

JASON A. BEYEA, MD, PhD
Neurotology Fellow, Department of Otolaryngology-Head and Neck Surgery, The Ohio State University, Columbus, Ohio

JOSEPH T. BREEN, MD
Otology/Neurotology Fellow, Department of Otolaryngology-Head and Neck Surgery, Baylor College of Medicine, Houston, Texas

MATTHEW L. CARLSON, MD
Assistant Professor, Department of Otolaryngology-Head and Neck Surgery, Mayo Clinic School of Medicine, Rochester, Minnesota

C. EDUARDO CORRALES, MD
Department of Otology, Neurotology and Skull Base Surgery, Division of Otolaryngology-Head and Neck Surgery, Brigham and Women's Hospital, Harvard Medical School, Boston, Massachusetts

NANCY FISCHBEIN, MD
Professor (By courtesy), Departments of Radiology, Otolaryngology-Head and Neck Surgery, Neurology, Neurosurgery, and Radiation Oncology, Stanford University Medical Center, Stanford, California

MICHAEL B. GLUTH, MD, FACS
Assistant Professor, Section of Otolaryngology-Head and Neck Surgery; Associate, Bloom Otopathology Laboratory; Director, Comprehensive Ear and Hearing Center, University of Chicago Medicine and Biological Sciences, Chicago, Illinois

RICHARD K. GURGEL, MD
Division of Otolaryngology, University of Utah, Salt Lake City, Utah

DAVID S. HAYNES, MD, FACS
Professor, Department of Otolaryngology-Head and Neck Surgery, Vanderbilt University, Nashville, Tennessee

BRANDON ISAACSON, MD, FACS
Co-Director of the Comprehensive Skull Base Program; Associate Professor, Department of Otolaryngology-Head and Neck Surgery, University of Texas Southwestern Medical Center, Dallas, Texas

ROBERT K. JACKLER, MD
Sewall Professor and Chair, Division of Otolaryngology-Head & Neck Surgery, Stanford University School of Medicine, Stanford, California

SHIRA KOSS, MD
Department of Otolaryngology-Head and Neck Surgery, The New York Eye and Ear Infirmary, New York, New York

NAUMAN F. MANZOOR, MD
Resident, Ear, Nose, and Throat Institute, University Hospitals Case Medical Center, Case Western Reserve University School of Medicine, Cleveland, Ohio

CLIFF A. MEGERIAN, MD, FACS
Julius W. McCall Professor and Chairman, Department of Otolaryngology-Head and Neck Surgery; Richard and Patricia Pogue Endowed Chair; Director, Ear, Nose, and Throat Institute, University Hospitals Case Medical Center, Case Western Reserve University School of Medicine, Cleveland, Ohio

AARON C. MOBERLY, MD
Assistant Professor, Department of Otolaryngology-Head and Neck Surgery, The Ohio State University, Columbus, Ohio

STANLEY PELOSI, MD
Assistant Professor, Department of Otolaryngology-Head and Neck Surgery, Thomas Jefferson University, Philadelphia, Pennsylvania

MAROUN T. SEMAAN, MD, FACS
Director, Otology, Neurotology, and Balance Disorders; Associate Professor, Department of Otolaryngology-Head and Neck Surgery, Ear, Nose, and Throat Institute, University Hospitals Case Medical Center, Case Western Reserve University School of Medicine, Cleveland, Ohio

ALEX D. SWEENEY, MD
Neurotology Fellow, Department of Otolaryngology-Head and Neck Surgery, Vanderbilt University, Nashville, Tennessee

ANDREW J. THOMAS, MD
Division of Otolaryngology, University of Utah, Salt Lake City, Utah

JEFFREY T. VRABEC, MD
Professor, Department of Otolaryngology-Head and Neck Surgery, Baylor College of Medicine, Houston, Texas

GEORGE B. WANNA, MD, FACS
Associate Professor, Department of Otolaryngology-Head and Neck Surgery, Division of Otology–Neurotology & Skull Base Surgery; Co-Director, Neurotology Fellowship Program; Vanderbilt University, Nashville, Tennessee

CAMERON C. WICK, MD
Chief Resident, Ear, Nose, and Throat Institute, University Hospitals Case Medical Center, Case Western Reserve University School of Medicine, Cleveland, Ohio

RICHARD H. WIGGINS III, MD
Division of Otolaryngology, University of Utah, Salt Lake City, Utah

Contents

Preface: Tumors of the Ear and Lateral Skull Base: Part I   xiii

George B. Wanna and Matthew L. Carlson

Early Practice: Neurotology   257

Joseph T. Breen and Jeffrey T. Vrabec

> Besides technical and surgical proficiency, some of the most important skills for a young Neurotologist to refine include communication and critical thinking abilities. This Early Practice article provides perspectives on common challenges and career development from a current Neurotology fellow and his mentor.

Imaging Innovations in Temporal Bone Disorders   263

C. Eduardo Corrales, Nancy Fischbein, and Robert K. Jackler

> The development of new imaging techniques coupled with new treatment algorithms has created new possibilities in treating temporal bone diseases. This article provides an overview of recent imaging innovations that can be applied to temporal bone diseases. Topics covered include the role of magnetic resonance (MR) diffusion-weighted imaging in cholesteatomas and skull base epidermoids, whole-body molecular imaging in paragangliomas of the jugular foramen, and MR arterial spin labeling perfusion for dural arteriovenous fistulas and arteriovenous malformations.

Squamous Cell Carcinoma of the Temporal Bone   281

Jason A. Beyea and Aaron C. Moberly

> Temporal bone malignancy presents a significant clinical challenge for the otolaryngologist. This article provides an overview of squamous cell carcinoma of the temporal bone, including clinical presentation, diagnosis, staging, treatment, and prognosis. As demonstrated in this case study, the prognosis for patients with advanced-stage temporal bone malignancy is poor, even with maximal therapy.

Glomus Tympanicum Tumors   293

Alex D. Sweeney, Matthew L. Carlson, George B. Wanna, and Marc L. Bennett

 Videos of the pulsation of a temporal bone paraganglioma behind an intact tympanic membrane and stepwise, microsurgical resection of an anteriorly based glomus tympanicum accompany this article

> Glomus tympanicum (GT) tumors are benign arising from paraganglion cells of the tympanic plexus in the middle ear. Although surgical resection remains the best option for definitive treatment of these tumors, the diagnostic and management algorithms have evolved considerably with the introduction of high-resolution computed tomography, MRI, and genetic testing.

Adenomatous Tumors of the Middle Ear   305

Stanley Pelosi and Shira Koss

Adenomatous tumors are an uncommon cause of a middle ear mass. Clinical findings may be nonspecific, leading to difficulties in differentiation from other middle ear tumors. Controversy also exists whether to classify middle ear adenoma and carcinoid as separate neoplasms, or alternatively within a spectrum of the same pathologic entity. Most adenomatous middle ear tumors are indolent in behavior, with a benign histologic appearance and slowly progressive growth. The mainstay of treatment is complete surgical resection, which affords the greatest likelihood of cure.

Endolymphatic Sac Tumors   317

Cameron C. Wick, Nauman F. Manzoor, Maroun T. Semaan, and Cliff A. Megerian

Endolymphatic sac tumors (ELST) are slow-growing, locally aggressive, low-grade malignancies that originate from the epithelium of the endolymphatic duct and sac. ELST often present with sensorineural hearing loss, tinnitus, and vertigo, which may mimic Meniere disease. Large tumors may present with additional cranial neuropathies. Management is primarily via microsurgical excision. Radiation therapy has a limited role for residual or unresectable disease. Early detection may enable hearing preservation techniques. ELST have an association with von Hippel–Lindau disease.

Contemporary Management of Jugular Paragangliomas   331

George B. Wanna, Alex D. Sweeney, David S. Haynes, and Matthew L. Carlson

Jugular paragangliomas are generally benign slow-growing tumors that can cause pulsatile tinnitus, hearing loss, and cranial nerves neuropathy. Progressive growth can also lead to intracranial extension. Historically, the treatment of choice for these lesions has been gross total resection. However, over the last 15 years, many groups have adopted less invasive management strategies including stereotactic radiation therapy, subtotal resection, and primary observation in order to reduce treatment-associated morbidity. The focus of this article is to review the modern management of jugular paraganglioma, highlighting the evolving treatment paradigm at the Otology Group of Vanderbilt.

Nonparaganglioma Jugular Foramen Tumors   343

Andrew J. Thomas, Richard H. Wiggins III, and Richard K. Gurgel

This article discusses the epidemiology, presentation, and diagnostic work-up of nonparaganglioma jugular foramen tumors, and the management options and predicted outcomes. Paragangliomas are the most common jugular foramen tumors, but other nonparagangliomas are important to consider in a differential for jugular foramen tumors. This article specifically focuses on jugular foramen schwannomas, meningiomas, metastatic disease, and regional pathologies that may extend to the jugular foramen, such as endolymphatic sac tumors, chordomas, and chondrosarcomas. Operative approaches to these tumors are also reviewed.

Cholesterol Granuloma and Other Petrous Apex Lesions   361

Brandon Isaacson

> This article presents the latest information on the presentation, diagnosis, imaging characteristics, management, and outcomes for petrous apex cholesterol granulomas. An in-depth review of the pathophysiology and surgical approaches is presented along with a summary of other petrous apex lesions and their imaging characteristics.

Rhabdomyosarcoma and Other Pediatric Temporal Bone Malignancies   375

Michael B. Gluth

> This article outlines the nature of temporal bone malignancy in children, particularly from the viewpoint of a surgeon. This article includes a synopsis of the presentation, workup, and management options for children affected by these uncommon tumors. Particular attention is given to rhabdomyosarcoma, including an update of modern staging, risk classification, and prognosis; however, a concise review of other forms of pediatric temporal bone cancer and an overview of surgical approaches available for treatment is undertaken as well.

Index   391

OTOLARYNGOLOGIC CLINICS OF NORTH AMERICA

FORTHCOMING ISSUES

June 2015
Tumors of the Ear and Lateral Skull Base, Part 2
George Wanna and Matthew Carlson, *Editors*

August 2015
Function Preservation in Laryngeal Cancer
Babak Sadoughi, *Editor*

October 2015
Medical and Surgical Complications in the Treatment of Chronic Rhinosinusitis
James A. Stankiewicz, *Editor*

December 2015
Hemostasis in Head and Neck Surgery
Carl P. Snyderman and Harshita Pant, *Editors*

RECENT ISSUES

February 2015
Pediatric Head and Neck Masses
John Maddalozzo and Jeffrey C. Rastatter, *Editors*

December 2014
Ear Implants
Colin Driscoll and Brian Neff, *Editors*

October 2014
Common ENT Disorders in Children
Charles Bower and Gresham Richter, *Editors*

August 2014
Thyroid Cancer: Current Diagnosis, Management, and Prognostication
Robert L. Witt, *Editor*

DOWNLOAD Free App!

Review Articles
THE CLINICS

NOW AVAILABLE FOR YOUR iPhone and iPad

Preface

Tumors of the Ear and Lateral Skull Base: Part I

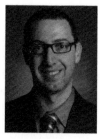 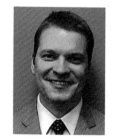

George B. Wanna, MD, FACS   Matthew L. Carlson, MD
Editors

Over the past 100 years, the evaluation and management of lateral skull-base tumors have evolved tremendously. While most pathology involving the temporal bone and cerebellopontine angle is histologically benign, significant morbidity may occur as a result of disease progression or treatment. At the turn of the twentieth century, mortality from cerebellopontine angle tumor extirpation exceeded 80% and invariably resulted in substantial cranial nerve morbidity in the small percentage of those that survived the perioperative window. As a result of refinements in diagnostic imaging, microsurgical techniques, and stereotactic radiation delivery, today disease and treatment-associated mortality approaches zero and the majority of patients receive durable tumor control and experience minimal neurologic morbidity. Recognizing the significant advantages of multidisciplinary care, most centers utilize the collective expertise of neurotologists, neurosurgeons, and radiation oncologists in the treatment of patients with lateral skull-base tumors.

It is a great honor and privilege to guest edit this important two-part issue of *Otolaryngologic Clinics of North America* titled "Tumors of the Ear and Lateral Skull Base." We were extremely fortunate to assemble a cadre of world-renowned experts to share their clinical insights and knowledge regarding the complex and evolving treatment of lateral skull-base disease. Part 1 is primarily dedicated to temporal bone tumors, covering innovative imaging techniques, external auditory canal malignancy, glomus tympanicum, adenomatous tumors of the middle ear, endolymphatic sac tumors, glomus jugulare, jugular foramen meningioma and schwannoma, cholesterol granuloma, and pediatric temporal bone malignancies. We extend our sincerest gratitude to each

Otolaryngol Clin N Am 48 (2015) xiii–xiv
http://dx.doi.org/10.1016/j.otc.2015.01.001
0030-6665/15/$ – see front matter © 2015 Published by Elsevier Inc.

oto.theclinics.com

contributing author for dedicating a significant amount of time and effort towards the completion of this comprehensive two-part issue.

George B. Wanna, MD, FACS
Division of Otology–Neurotology & Skull Base Surgery
Neurotology Fellowship Program
The Otology Group of Vanderbilt
Vanderbilt University Medical Center
1215 21st Avenue South
7209 Medical Center East, South Tower
Nashville, TN 37232, USA

Matthew L. Carlson, MD
Division of Otology–Neurotology & Skull Base Surgery
Mayo Clinic
Gonda Building, 12S-ENT
200 First Street
Rochester, MN 55905, USA

E-mail addresses:
george.wanna@vanderbilt.edu (G.B. Wanna)
carlson.matthew@mayo.edu (M.L. Carlson)

Early Practice: Neurotology

Joseph T. Breen, MD*, Jeffrey T. Vrabec, MD

KEYWORDS

- Practice • Professionalism • Education • Training • Career • Leadership
- Mentoring

KEY POINTS

- Tumors of the ear and temporal bone present numerous treatment challenges for all surgeons, particularly those in the early stages of their careers.
- Although the trainee will tend to focus on learning technical and surgical details, some of the most important skills for a young neurotologist to refine include communication and critical thinking abilities.
- Critical analysis of the literature and one's own results will lead to continuous improvement and a rewarding career.

INTRODUCTION

As a distinct medical and surgical specialty, neurotology is still young. The work of pioneering individuals in the mid-20th century laid the groundwork for the modern treatment of temporal bone and cerebellopontine angle tumors. Despite the relatively short history of neurotology, management strategies for these tumors have evolved significantly because of recent technological advances, refinements in surgical techniques, and growing knowledge of the natural history of lateral skull base diseases.

Young surgeons in their final years of residency and fellowship, as well as those just beginning in independent practice, face the formidable challenge of accumulating the necessary knowledge for comprehensive management of skull base tumors. Even at high-volume academic medical centers, trainees may only encounter a handful of examples of some of the diseases neurotologists are called upon to treat. With a relatively small volume of personal experience to draw from, an ever-growing body of literature, increasingly high expectations from patients and payers, and an inherently challenging set of diseases to treat, young neurotologists may find themselves overwhelmed in early stages of their career.

This *Early Practice* article, a feature new to the *Clinics*, is intended to be a collection of insights and observations that residents, fellows, and recent graduates might find

Department of Otolaryngology - Head and Neck Surgery, Baylor College of Medicine, Houston, TX, USA
* Corresponding author. Department of Otolaryngology - Head and Neck Surgery, Baylor College of Medicine, 6550 Fannin Suite 1727, Houston, TX 77030.
E-mail address: jbreen@bcm.edu

Otolaryngol Clin N Am 48 (2015) 257–262
http://dx.doi.org/10.1016/j.otc.2014.12.001
0030-6665/15/$ – see front matter © 2015 Elsevier Inc. All rights reserved.

useful as they transition into practice. The details of tumor-specific patient management will be left to those colleagues who are contributing to this 2-part series. Instead, perspectives will be provided by a current neurotology fellow (JTB) and his mentor (JTV) in a discussion about the everyday challenges faced by practicing lateral skull base surgeons. Out of decades of experience, the mentor has identified 6 key skills and qualities a successful neurotologist must exhibit. These items will be examined from the perspective of a surgeon just beginning his or her career as well as that of a seasoned veteran.

RESPONSIBILITY
Breen

As surgeons and physicians, we are privileged to care for our patients. For neurotologists, this privilege is coupled to the expectation that we are ready to provide the highest level of care for patients with challenging problems. Medicine has become a profession far too complex for any practitioner to be expected to have comprehensive knowledge of all disease. When deciding to become a subspecialist, however, the trainee has committed himself or herself to an intense course of study in his or her chosen field.

Opinions on optimal treatment may vary, particularly with the relatively rare diseases treated by neurotologists, but appropriate decisions simply cannot be made without a comprehensive fund of knowledge. There is no substitute for reading the relevant literature, studying in the temporal bone laboratory, and participating in the care of patients treated by our mentors. Particularly in an era of increasing trainee numbers, decreasing surgical case numbers, and duty hour restrictions, every patient encounter is one that demands the full attention of the trainee to maximize the learning experience. The lucky few who have the opportunity to train with masters in this field have a responsibility to become experts. This cannot happen if a strong foundation is not laid by many hours of hard work during the training years.

Vrabec

It is difficult for the trainee to fully understand the burden of responsibility that comes with independent practice, because there is always a faculty member serving as the final decision maker. However, this lesson is rapidly learned. No matter how broad an experience a trainee receives, one can never see everything. There are usually a few moments in the first few months of practice where a novel clinical problem or operative situation arises, and the new practitioner must respond. When the newly acquired knowledge and skills are challenged, the graduate understands the assumption of responsibility that comes with independent practice.

Even after decades of practice, clinical challenges continue to arise. This intellectual stimulation is one of the most rewarding aspects of the profession. It is unlikely that one will ever become bored with clinical or operative care. Responding to novel situations requires a broad perspective on the range of possible actions, anticipation of potential outcomes, consideration of comparable problems, and assigning probabilities of success to each available choice. The ultimate decision may be questioned by patients or colleagues. The ability to discuss the decision making logically and accurately and respond to criticism is the definition of the responsible physician.

COMMUNICATION
Breen

Even when caring for individuals with tumors of the ear and temporal bone, it is uncommon that the neurotologist is discussing matters of life and death with patients.

Rather, the patient and surgeon must both understand the relative weight that the patient places on morbidities (eg, hearing loss, disequilibrium, facial weakness, or lower cranial neuropathies) potentially associated with the disease or with treatment. To arrive at this mutual understanding, the patient must be given a clear and appropriately detailed explanation of his or her disease, the possible outcomes with treatment, and the expected outcome if the patient elects for no treatment at all. The perceptive surgeon will note the feedback from the patient to help him or her make a decision.

Having been trained in a medical culture where a strong emphasis is placed on patient autonomy, these statements seem self-evident to physicians of my generation. However, I have not uncommonly encountered the patient who simply will want to follow whatever treatment recommendation is provided, divorcing themselves from the decision-making process. It is just as important in these situations that all aspects of the patient's medical and social history be taken into account and that the patient understands the implications of the agreed-upon treatment.

Vrabec

No longer an intermediary, the new surgeon is the primary contact for all aspects of patient care and must develop and maintain excellent communication with patients, families, operating room personnel, and collaborating surgeons. Optimal outcomes are achieved when everyone has the same understanding of the proposed intervention, anticipated benefits, and possible risks. There are specific types of information for each group, such as postoperative instructions for the patient, sequence of interventions for the operating room personnel, and division of labor among surgeons.

Sometimes the information must be presented multiple times or in different levels of complexity for the understanding to develop. Ask questions and encourage dialogue to uncover misunderstandings prior to the intervention.

JUDGMENT
Breen

Residency and fellowship provide the building blocks for becoming an independent surgeon. These components include mastery of the physical examination, practice with surgical techniques, and recognition of common patterns of treatment. One learns how to overcome intraoperative challenges and accomplish surgical objectives as training progresses. However, the trainee often misses out on the crucial decision making that occurred before the patient arrived in the operating room.

When the resident or fellow is working under the guidance of an experienced and trusted mentor, he or she is reassured that the treatment plan is a sound one. As opportunities for independent decision making arise later in training, however, it becomes apparent that these decisions are rarely clear-cut. Uncertainty will surround decisions made early in practice, in particular. Some uncertainty must be accepted, but the early practitioner should learn to recognize situations warranting additional data or consultation from a more experienced colleague. Understanding one's own limitations and the limits of what is possible will lead to sound treatment decisions.

Vrabec

Training programs typically do an excellent job of teaching technique. The case volume and complexity are high, allowing frequent participation. Temporal bone laboratories are available, giving further opportunity to hone skills for lateral skull base approaches. Because every patient is different, the operative plan should anticipate the anatomic limitations of tumor resection and define an achievable objective. Review of preoperative imaging with radiology colleagues helps to clarify any indistinct tumor margins and adjacent structures. If total excision will not be possible without significant potential morbidity, then the benefit to the patient of a subtotal resection should be clear. Because many of the tumors treated by the neurotologist are benign, less invasive means for palliation have to be presented in detail.

Even the best operative plan may have to be altered because of intraoperative circumstances. When unforeseen obstacles arise, the surgeon must be flexible and accept a different outcome than originally proposed, such as a requirement for an unplanned second-stage procedure. First, do no harm. The experienced surgeon understands the limitations of operative intervention.

With experience, the surgeon may better determine the impact of the disease on an individual patient. Making the tumor go away does not always lead to improvement in the patient's quality of life. Rather, the surgeon must consider how the alteration in hearing or balance will benefit the patient and whether avoidance of future problems is sufficient to assume the risks of intervention. The patient may have a vastly different perspective than the surgeon, such as the assessment of facial function. The surgeon may consider mild weakness a successful outcome, but the patient may not. There have to be realistic expectations for both patient and surgeon. Promising perfection and delivering less will certainly lead to dissatisfied patients.

EFFICIENCY
Breen

A difficult but quickly performed procedure by an experienced attending surgeon never fails to impress the trainee. It is not until the later years of training, however, that some perspective is gained on what makes an expeditious surgery. Certainly it is not the speed at which the surgeon's hands move; if anything, some of the most technically impressive surgeons I've seen tend to transition to a slow and precise mode during tumor dissection or other key portions of cases. Part of the improvement comes from technical advances, such as increased dexterity with practice, understanding of anatomy, and experience in tissue handling. A significant factor separating the novice from the master, however, is how far in advance one is thinking while performing each step of an operation. The trainee may only be able to think about the immediate task at hand, not always having an appreciation of how the current surgical maneuver is influencing the next or the overall goals of the operation. The master makes every move with purpose, leverages his or her operating room team to maximum effect, and is constantly thinking several steps ahead of where the operation presently stands. It is from these gains in efficiency that not only surgical speed, but also safety and effectiveness, improve with time.

Vrabec

Surgical volume is usually low in the first few years of practice, emphasizing the need to seek opportunities to maintain and refine technical skills. Mastery of approaches improves efficiency and time management. The approach is the most predictable portion of the procedure and often proceeds through relatively normal anatomy. If too much time is spent on the preliminary steps, the more time-consuming and technically challenging portions of the case are delayed. The surgeon becomes more fatigued, and dedicated support personnel may be relieved by less specialized individuals on the late shift, making the dissection even more difficult.

Learning to work with other surgeons is a training process for all. The strengths and weaknesses of each may not be evident until well into the procedure as one struggles with a step one thought the other surgeon would do. This type of teamwork requires a number of cases together, although the process is enhanced by the experience of either individual. Thus, the new neurotologist will improve faster by working with an experienced neurosurgeon and vice versa. Expect cases to take much longer in early practice and schedule operating room time accordingly.

CRITICAL ANALYSIS
Breen

Without years of personal experience to help guide decision making, the journeyman surgeon turns to the literature and to seasoned mentors. However, tried-and-true algorithms for management of most lateral skull base tumors are essentially nonexistent. Recommendations and suggestions abound, but consensus is rarely reached. Treatment strategies used by prominent surgeons, institutions, or training lineages may come to the forefront, but those surgeons' equally prominent colleagues from other schools of thought might take a different approach. Based on the present data and our understanding of the natural history of rare skull base tumors, various approaches may be equally reasonable.

As a result, our direct mentors will strongly influence our initial practice patterns. However, a critical eye is needed to distinguish between decisions based on strong evidence, decisions made "because it's always been done that way," and those that lie somewhere between. If one is expected to not just maintain the field, but improve it, one must question authority to some degree.

Vrabec

Was the desired outcome achieved? If so, the surgeon reaps praise from grateful patients. If not, then criticism is expected. It is natural to prefer to remember the successes; however, the greater learning opportunity is gained through critical analysis of unfavorable results. Was the cause for the poor outcome due to technique, decision making, improper planning, inadequate knowledge or poor communication? Focusing on these issues consistently is a good way to enhance future results.

The medical literature defines outcomes from the surgeon's perspective (no residual tumor, an air bone gap <20 dB, a healed tympanic membrane). Patients have different opinions (taste change, pain or paresthesia of the operative site, change in appearance). The patient's rating systems are not uniform. What is deemed acceptable morbidity by 1 patient may be devastating to another. Listening to the results from the patient perspective improves preoperative counseling. Discussion of potential complications alerts the surgeon to the patient's key concerns.

It is not uncommon to read or listen to presentations boasting of perfect outcomes, implying that the less successful are inferior practitioners. But are the results confirmed by other surgeons? The "perfect" surgeons are lacking insight of the patient's experience and can therefore never improve. It is important to listen to the patients and focus on refining interventions for their benefit.

LIFETIME LEARNING
Breen

If what I knew about neurotology was confined to what my mentors directly taught me, my knowledge base would certainly be lacking. This is not to disparage my mentors, but rather to highlight the fact that teaching is not always a direct transfer of knowledge. What one learns from the best teachers is a framework for thinking and approaching problems that can be applied to future challenges. The current generation of leaders in neurotology may not have trained at a time when cochlear implantation was particularly common or when superior semicircular canal dehiscence was even a described entity, but these surgeons are looked to as authorities on such matters. Obviously, learning does not stop when residency or fellowship ends.

Vrabec

Medical knowledge is dynamic. Older literature must be interpreted within the context of available knowledge at the time it was written. Some things that were generally accepted 25 years ago are no longer true. The underlying pathophysiology of most neurotological disorders is not completely understood. Elements of practice are certain to change over time as new understandings of pathophysiology emerge. Not all advances can be confirmed with rigorous clinical trials. It is imperative to thoroughly study new developments to separate the publicity stunts from true advances.

SUMMARY

Much is expected of the neurotologist. The treatment of lateral skull base tumors involves a great deal of technical skill, knowledge, and decision-making ability. In addition, this work is often done in an academic environment, where the surgeon is also expected to be a leader, teacher, and scholar. These are intimidating challenges for the early practitioner. Many years of formal education provide a solid foundation, but learning and development must continue beyond the training years if a successful career is expected.

Imaging Innovations in Temporal Bone Disorders

C. Eduardo Corrales, MD[a], Nancy Fischbein, MD[b], Robert K. Jackler, MD[c],*

KEYWORDS

- Cholesteatoma • Diffusion-weighted imaging • Paraganglioma
- Whole-body molecular imaging • Dural arteriovenous fistula
- Arteriovenous malformation • Arterial spin labeling

KEY POINTS

- High-resolution computed tomography is a fast and dependable method for assessing temporal bone anatomy and planning surgical approach in cases of cholesteatoma.
- Diffusion-weighted MRI is likely to decrease the number of second-look surgeries, decreasing patient morbidity and surgical costs.
- Contrast-enhanced computed tomography of the skull base, MRI of the skull base and neck, and catheter angiography and embolization in the preoperative period are recommended for evaluation and management of jugular foramen paragangliomas.
- Arterial spin labeling (ASL) is an emerging noninvasive MRI procedure that does not require gadolinium-based contrast administration and is a useful diagnostic test for dural arteriovenous fistulas (DAVFs) and small arteriovenous malformations (AVMs) less than 2 cm.
- The absence of venous signal on ASL is a helpful predictor of the presence or absence of DAVF or AVM in patients with pulsatile tinnitus and no obvious vascular malformation on routine imaging studies.

INTRODUCTION

Important advances in diagnostic imaging of the temporal bone have been made in the past decade. The development of new imaging techniques coupled with new treatment algorithms has created new possibilities in treating temporal bone diseases. This article provides an overview of recent imaging innovations that can be applied to temporal bone diseases; it does not provide a comprehensive review of temporal

Disclosures: None.
[a] Department of Otology, Neurotology and Skull Base Surgery, Division of Otolaryngology-Head and Neck Surgery, Brigham and Women's Hospital, Harvard Medical School, 45 Francis Street, Boston, MA 02115, USA; [b] Departments of Radiology, Otolaryngology-Head and Neck Surgery, Neurology, Neurosurgery and Radiation Oncology, Stanford University Medical Center, 300 Pasteur Drive, Room S-047, Stanford, CA 94305, USA; [c] Division of Otolaryngology-Head & Neck Surgery, Stanford University School of Medicine, 801 Welch Road, Stanford, CA 94305, USA
* Corresponding author.
E-mail address: jackler@stanford.edu

Otolaryngol Clin N Am 48 (2015) 263–280
http://dx.doi.org/10.1016/j.otc.2014.12.002
0030-6665/15/$ – see front matter © 2015 Elsevier Inc. All rights reserved.

Abbreviations	
ASL	Arterial spin labeling
AVMs	Arteriovenous malformations
CBCT	Cone beam computed tomography
CT	Computed tomography
CTA	Computed tomography angiography
DAVFs	Dural arteriovenous fistulas
DOPA	Dihydroxyphenylalanine
DOTATATE	Tetraazacyclododecane tetraacetic acid-octreotate
DSA	Digital subtraction angiography
DTPA	Diethylenetriaminepentaacetic acid
DWI	Diffusion-weighted imaging
EPI	Echo-planar imaging
^{18}F-FDG	^{18}F-fluorodeoxyglucose
HRCT	High-resolution computed tomography
IV	Intravenous
MIBG	Metaiodobenzylguanidine
MR	Magnetic resonance
MRA	Magnetic resonance angiography
MRV	Magnetic resonance venography
NET	Neuroendocrine tumors
PGL-1	Paraganglioma syndrome 1

bone disorders and their imaging characteristics, because numerous excellent references already exist in textbooks and review articles.[1–4]

Topics covered in this article include imaging techniques for evaluation of cholesteatoma and epidermoids, with emphasis on the role of magnetic resonance (MR) diffusion-weighted imaging (DWI); imaging techniques for evaluation of skull base neuroendocrine tumors, including paragangliomas, with emphasis on whole-body molecular imaging; and MR arterial spin labeling (ASL) perfusion for dural arteriovenous fistulas (DAVFs) and arteriovenous malformations (AVMs).

Imaging Techniques for Evaluation of Cholesteatoma and Epidermoids

Since its introduction in the early 1980s, high-resolution computed tomography (HRCT) of the temporal bone has been the gold standard for imaging cholesteatoma.[5–7] HRCT now represents the preeminent modality for defining the bony anatomy of the temporal bone, as well as pathologic alterations in that anatomy caused by cholesteatoma. Although cholesteatoma is usually readily identified based on history and otoscopic examination, its presence and extent may not always be clear. This considerable unpredictability in size and extent of cholesteatoma can substantially affect surgical approach, expectations, and risk, as can the possible involvement of critical adjacent structures. Despite these strengths of HRCT, in postoperative ears, residual or recurrent cholesteatoma may be in areas concealed from direct inspection, leading to the necessity of second-look surgeries for complete evaluation, because HRCT cannot conclusively distinguish residual or recurrent disease from fluid and granulation tissue, which have similar density.

Because HRCT is limited in its ability to differentiate among soft tissue densities in the temporal bone, the addition of MRI, with its superior soft tissue contrast, has been valuable in the temporal bone. The recent development and refinements of diffusion-weighted MRI (DW-MRI) have contributed significantly in this regard, allowing accurate identification of the presence of small foci of keratin debris that would otherwise be impossible to differentiate from fluid, edematous mucosa, and/or granulation tissue on routine MR sequences and HRCT. In this way, the selective use of HRCT and DW-MRI can provide complementary information that can guide otologic surgeons in the management of cholesteatoma.

The strength of HRCT is its capacity to image bone. A cholesteatoma appears as a soft tissue mass, usually occurring in pneumatized regions of the temporal bone. The normal aeration is lost and the surrounding bone often shows evidence of erosion with smooth or scalloped margins. Adjacent ossicles may be absent, eroded, or demineralized. The scutum is often eroded, revealing the pathway of ingrowth of epithelium from the pars flaccida into the epitympanum (**Fig. 1**). HRCT is also useful in recognizing the geometry and location of adjacent vital structures. The bony labyrinth, facial nerve canal, tegmen, sigmoid plate, and carotid canal can all be well seen on HRCT. A careful study of the HRCT can also reveal anatomic variations that may affect surgery, such as dehiscence of the facial nerve canal. Similarly, loss of the normal bone overlying any of these structures may give a valuable warning of involvement by cholesteatoma.

When ossicular or mastoid bony erosion is seen in association with a soft tissue mass, HRCT can distinguish cholesteatoma with specificity between 80% and 90%.[8,9] In the postoperative period, HRCT has a high negative predictive value when it shows a well-aerated middle ear with no evidence of soft tissue densities.[8,10,11] However, HRCT has proved unreliable in differentiating residual or recurrent cholesteatoma from granulation tissue, cholesterol granuloma, mucosal edema, fibrosis, scar tissue, or fluid.[10,12,13] However, in patients who have undergone previous tympanomastoidectomy, the relevance of bony erosion is lost because it is difficult or impossible to differentiate surgical changes from pathologic bony destruction caused by cholesteatoma. In this setting, HRCT has a sensitivity of 43%, specificity of 42% to 51%, and a predictive value of 28% in detecting residual or recurrent cholesteatoma.[13,14]

The introduction of in-office cone beam computed tomography (CBCT) imaging has made imaging for cholesteatoma more convenient and accessible.[15] As a result of their favorable radiation safety profile and compact size, CBCT scanners can be assembled in clinic rooms with often minimal requirements for specialized shielding.

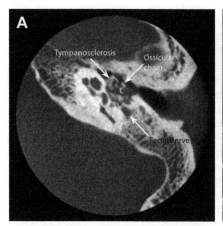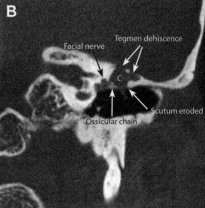

Fig. 1. HRCT of a patient with left cholesteatoma. Axial (A) view shows a sclerotic mastoid with an erosive cholesteatoma (c) There is tympanosclerosis medial to the ossicular chain. Coronal (B) view shows typical imaging features, including cholesteatoma (c) showing scalloped edges, scutum erosion, and a demineralized/eroded ossicular chain. The tegmen is dehiscent and low lying, making surgical access challenging. The facial nerve canal is shown to be dehiscent adjacent to the oval window on the coronal image.

In CBCT scanners, the x-ray beam forms a cone-shaped geometry between the imaging source (apex of the cone) and the detector (base of the cone). In contrast, conventional scanners have a fan-beam geometry.[16] The radiation dose of these scans is reported to be 60% of a conventional computed tomography (CT) scanner when evaluating middle ear structures,[16–18] but middle and inner ear bony structures are seen equally well in CBCT and conventional HRCT scanners.[17] One disadvantage of in-office CBCT is the limited anatomic coverage, which means inner ear or more distal disorders in the mastoid may be missed. An additional CBCT disadvantage is the lack of any soft tissue contrast, and these scanners are typically used only to assess bony anatomy. A general disadvantage of both HRCT and CBCT is their use of ionizing radiation, and hence their intrinsic potential for inducing malignancy.[19,20] Therefore, clinicians must always be judicious in their use, particularly in children who may be sensitive to cumulative radiation effects.

MRI

Although MRI cannot provide a map of the bony geometric framework of the temporal bone for surgical planning, selected MRI techniques can provide valuable information regarding the presence, size, and approximate location of cholesteatoma that may not be available on HRCT imaging. MRI also has the advantage of not requiring exposure to radiation, although it does require longer acquisition times compared with HRCT, and the need for immobilization may make it difficult to obtain in young children.

On conventional MRI sequences, cholesteatomas and epidermoids appear dark on T1-weighted images, bright on T2-weighted images, and do not enhance with intravenous contrast unless acute infection results in rim enhancement. These signal characteristics render them difficult to distinguish from much of the other soft tissue present in a chronic ear condition unless they are large. One mechanism to circumvent this limitation has been the use of delayed-contrast techniques. Delayed-contrast MRI has been used to better detect recurrent cholesteatoma by taking advantage of the fact that other tissue, such as fibrosis or granulation tissue, often takes up more contrast given sufficient time,[21–24] whereas cholesteatomas do not. In this technique, T1 images are obtained 30 to 45 minutes after intravenous (IV) paramagnetic contrast administration (gadolinium), which results in enhancement of inflammatory mucosa, granulation tissue, scar, or fibrosis. Absence of contrast enhancement in a lesion suggests cholesteatoma. De Foer and colleagues[23] reported sensitivity and specificity for delayed-contrast MRI in detecting cholesteatoma as 56.7% and 67.6% respectively. Overall positive predictive value was 88% and negative predictive value was 27% in the population studied. Disadvantages of using delayed-contrast MRI are (1) the cost and potential morbidity associated with the need for IV contrast; (2) retained secretions, silicone/plastic (Silastic [Dow Corning, MI]) sheets, and calcified scars can mimic nonperfused cholesteatoma; (3) early acquisition of images may lead to false-positives; (4) this technique cannot detect cholesteatomas smaller than 3 mm; (5) it is difficult for scheduling purposes to keep an MR scanner available if immediate and delayed scans are both acquired; and (6) sedation or general anesthesia is required for children because of the prolonged time required for image acquisition. As a result of these limitations, delayed-contrast MRI for detecting residual or recurrent cholesteatoma has never caught on and is not routinely used in most practices.

However, over the last decade the use of diffusion-weighted sequences has provided considerable improvement in the diagnosis of cholesteatoma and skull base epidermoids, and this sequence is now considered an important component of the MRI assessment for both diseases. DWI relies on the principles of molecular diffusion or brownian motion.[25] Molecular diffusion refers to the haphazard movement of water molecules, which is restricted in certain pathologic conditions, including in the presence of organized keratin debris as seen in both cholesteatoma and epidermoids.[26] In regions where the diffusion of water is impeded or restricted, there is less dephasing of protons and more signal is retained, and hence the tissue with restricted diffusion is seen as bright on the diffusion-weighted image.[10,25] The keratin debris associated with cholesteatomas and epidermoids restricts water diffusion, and this leads to a high signal intensity in this material on DWI compared with brain or other surrounding soft tissues. Granulation tissue, fibrosis, and mucosal edema are less restricting of water motion and do not lead to high signal on DWI.

Two broad categories of DWI algorithms can be used for initial evaluation of cholesteatoma and epidermoids, or detection of residual or recurrent cholesteatoma: echo-planar and non–echo-planar DW-MRI. The first algorithm developed was echo-planar DWI, and many articles have described its use in detecting cholesteatomas.[12,21–35] Echo-planar imaging (EPI)–based methods are fast and reliable, but they produce considerable distortion at the skull base and temporal bone related to the numerous interfaces among air, bone, and soft tissue, and to the inhomogeneity of the magnetic field that results from these interfaces, as discussed in more detail later. Non-EPI DW methods are typically either single-shot turbo-spin echo sequences (half Fourier acquisition single-shot turbo-spin echo [HASTE; Siemens Systems, Germany]) or multishot turbo-spin echo sequences (periodically rotated overlapping parallel lines with enhanced reconstruction [PROPELLER]; BLADE [Siemens Systems, Germany]), and they are less subject to distortion at the skull base.

As mentioned earlier, EPI DWI is subject to artifacts at the interfaces between tissues, especially when air or bone is adjacent to soft tissue. These magnetic susceptibility artifacts relate to local magnetic field inhomogeneities caused by tissues of markedly different composition; they can also occur in the vicinity of metallic foreign bodies, such as surgical clips or staples, or dental work. However, the mastoid and middle ear produce susceptibility artifacts caused by natural air-bone interfaces, and this causes image distortion. Multiple studies have shown the inability of EPI DWI to detect cholesteatomas smaller than 5 mm.[10] Studies have also shown newer, non-EPI DWI methods to be superior to EPI DWI in detecting recurrent or residual cholesteatoma,[26,29,34] and thus non-EPI DWI has become the standard for MRI imaging of cholesteatoma. Skull base epidermoids located in the cerebello-pontine angle (CPA) and petroclival junction, have less susceptibility artifacts.

Various studies,[26,28,29,34] including a recent meta-analysis,[32] have evaluated DW-MRI for the detection of residual and recurrent cholesteatomas. In the meta-analysis, the overall sensitivity of this imaging modality was 94% with a specificity of 94%. Most of the false-negatives reported were caused by cholesteatoma pearls less than 3 mm in size. False-positives reported in this study were caused by susceptibility artifacts, cholesterol granuloma, abscess, or bone powder; in some of these cases the image showed a true disorder, but this disorder was not necessarily cholesteatoma.

Although MRI can be helpful in imaging of cholesteatoma under specific circumstances, the cost of MRI is approximately double that of HRCT.[36] Although clinicians should consider this additional economic impact, the benefits gained in selected patients by avoiding needless surgery, or by preventing a delay in diagnosis, can potentially justify its use on economic grounds.

INDICATIONS FOR IMAGING IN CHOLESTEATOMA AND EPIDERMOIDS

Experts may disagree about the indications for imaging in cholesteatoma and about the extent to which it assists in treatment decisions.[37] Some otologists routinely obtain imaging whenever cholesteatoma is seen or suspected, whereas others use imaging infrequently. Most agree that imaging is indicated in revision cases and those with intracranial or intratemporal complications. Surgeons should carefully consider the benefits they receive from imaging in their own practices, and they should regularly reevaluate imaging indications and referrals as they gain experience and perhaps modify their surgical techniques accordingly. Surgeons should also be diligent about reviewing imaging studies themselves, because even the best radiology report rarely conveys all the subtleties that may affect surgery.

For lesions located in the skull base, such as epidermoids, imaging is routinely obtained.

Preoperative Assessment

The benefits of being aware of potential challenges and of having a CT-based guide for surgical planning are particularly helpful in teaching settings, so that expectations for the case can be reviewed preoperatively. Similarly, HRCT can be helpful before revision surgery, especially when the surgeon did not perform the initial procedure. In revision cases, anatomy may be considerably altered, limiting the utility of normal surgical landmarks and presenting unexpected challenges.

HRCT can reveal specific patterns of pneumatization and aeration or variability in the position of the sigmoid sinus or tegmen, which may affect surgical access to the disorder. Is a mastoidectomy needed, or can the disease be adequately accessed via a transcanal approach? Is there likely to be adequate space to access disease with the canal wall left up, or is the mastoid sclerotic and contracted, warranting a canal-wall-down procedure? Erosion of the Fallopian canal may be suggested, as can exposure of the carotid artery or jugular bulb, and these findings are important alerts to potential hazards during dissection. Some labyrinthine fistulae are clinically silent,[38] as are almost all facial nerve canal erosions, thus preoperative knowledge of these findings may alert the surgeon to areas that warrant extra intraoperative care and attention. Although the ossicles are difficult to assess completely, obvious ossicular abnormalities may predict the need for ossicular reconstruction. HRCT can also show unexpected and potentially unrelated anatomic variations such as anomalous facial nerve patterns.[39]

Despite MRI's superior ability to identify cholesteatoma and differentiate it from other soft tissues, it is seldom helpful in the preoperative setting in primary cases unless there is a question about the preoperative diagnosis of cholesteatoma; in these cases, DW-MRI can provide additional information when clinical information is limited or the otoscopic examination is inconclusive. However, most of the time the diagnosis is not in doubt and HRCT is superior in providing information on relevant anatomic geometry. DW-MRI becomes considerably more useful in assessing the potential for postoperative recurrence of disease. In such cases, cholesteatoma may appear in areas inaccessible to clinical otomicroscopy or in unexpected areas, including the mastoid cavity, deep to reconstructive materials, and growing around adjacent structures where the furthest extent of cholesteatoma may have been missed on the primary procedure (**Fig. 2**). DW-MRI images must be interpreted in conjunction with other MRI sequences, because not all high-signal-intensity tissue on DW-MRI is cholesteatoma. In these cases, the use of other MRI sequences may be useful to predict an alternative diagnosis such as cholesterol granuloma, and to provide the surgeon and patient with expectations for treatment.

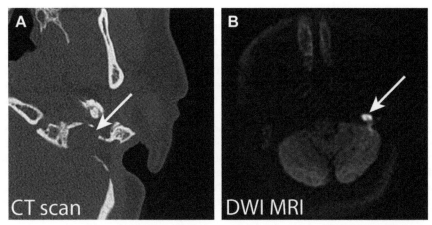

Fig. 2. Recurrent cholesteatoma (*arrow*) eroding the retrofacial air cells 25 years following a prior canal-wall-up tympanomastoidectomy. The patient's tympanic cavity showed no evidence of disease on otoscopy. (*A*) HRCT shows a nonspecific erosive soft tissue lesion with loss of bone over the sigmoid sinus and posterior fossa dura. (*B*) DWI-MRI shows focal high signal associated with the lesion, consistent with recurrent cholesteatoma (*arrow*).

Similarly, for epidermoids of the skull base, DWI-MRI is an extremely useful sequence to differentiate from arachnoid cysts (**Fig. 3**).

Postoperative Surveillance

It is compelling to look for alternatives to second-look surgery. If HRCT shows no abnormal soft tissue at 6 or 9 months following the initial stage, clinicians may be comfortable holding off on a second look.[8,10,11,37] However, it is rare that an HRCT study shows no nonspecific, potentially suspicious soft tissue. Also, in an early postoperative ear, bone erosion cannot be used to help differentiate the soft tissue from scar, fluid, or edema, and this is likely the situation in which DW-MRI is most useful in assessing cholesteatoma.

If postoperative imaging is done too early, false-negative DW-MRI may result. However, after 9 to 12 months, most persistent cholesteatomas are larger than 3 mm and

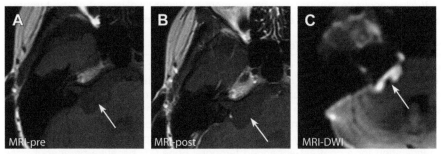

Fig. 3. Large epidermoid of the right cerebellopontine angle. (*A*) Axial T1-weighted image shows the lesion (*arrow*) to be of low signal intensity. (*B*) Axial postgadolinium T1-weighted image shows no enhancement of this lesion (*arrow*). From these sequences, it is nearly impossible to differentiate between an arachnoid cyst and an epidermoid. (*C*) Axial diffusion-weighted image shows a markedly increased signal intensity of the lesion (*arrow*), consistent with reduced diffusion, and thus an epidermoid.

therefore should be apparent on correctly performed DW-MRI.[26,28,29,32,34] A negative DW-MRI study may avoid the expense and morbidity associated with a negative second look. The surgeon needs to make the judgment regarding repeat surgery or imaging follow-up based on the likely area of involvement as to whether a recurrence of 3 mm or greater is unacceptably large. In some areas, such at the mastoid cavity, a recurrent lesion of this size can usually be readily resected. In other areas, such as the sinus tympani or on the stapes footplate, a cholesteatoma of 3 mm may present a greater surgical challenge. If this is the case, then foregoing imaging and proceeding directly to a second-look procedure is reasonable. If a DW-MRI study is negative at 9 to 12 months postoperatively, the surgeon should use clinical judgment as to whether another scan is needed at a later date. In routine cases, a single postoperative scan at 9 to 12 months may be sufficient, and the patient can be followed clinically. However, if there is concern for persistence in areas that are inherently more difficult to assess, such as the jugular foramen or petrous apex, then another scan obtained a year later is a reasonable option.

Cholesteatoma Complications

In patients with complications of cholesteatoma, imaging is almost always indicated.[21,34,40,41] MRI is well suited for defining intracranial complications such as brain abscess or epidural abscess, or sinus thrombosis, although contrast-enhanced CT can also be informative and is indicated if there are contraindications to MRI. MR venography (MRV) or CT venography may be helpful to evaluate for septic sigmoid thrombosis. In the setting of complications, clinicians may wish to obtain both HRCT and MRI studies, because each may offer valuable insights into diagnostic and therapeutic implications.

WHOLE-BODY MOLECULAR IMAGING IN PARAGANGLIOMAS OF THE JUGULAR FORAMEN

The most common paraganglioma in the head and neck region is the carotid body tumor, followed by paraganglioma of the jugular bulb (jugulare), middle ear (tympanicum), and vagal paragangliomas.[42] Tympanic paragangliomas are the most common primary neoplasms of the middle ear[43] and jugular paragangliomas are the most common tumors of the jugular foramen.[44] The most common symptoms for both jugular and tympanic paragangliomas are pulsatile tinnitus and hearing loss.[43,45–48] CT and MRI allow accurate preoperative assessment of tumor involvement of the temporal bone and skull base, as well as an evaluation for intracranial extension.

High-resolution Computed Tomography

Thin-section HRCT scan (<1 mm) in both axial and direct planes or, more commonly, reconstructed coronal plane is the imaging modality of choice to assess for temporal bone involvement and to visualize bony structures and tumor extension (**Fig. 4**). HRCT scan is useful to discriminate between paragangliomas that arise from the middle ear (tympanic) and paragangliomas arising from the jugular bulb (jugular). Although temporal bone HRCT is typically done without contrast, suspicion of a vascular mass is an indication for a contrast-enhanced temporal bone CT, because paragangliomas enhance intensely postcontrast. The characteristic location, pattern of bone erosion, and intense enhancement generally allow paragangliomas to be differentiated from most benign and malignant tumors of the skull base. In patients with pulsatile tinnitus and a vascular middle ear mass, HRCT helps to easily differentiate among paraganglioma, aberrant internal carotid artery, and a dehiscent jugular bulb,[49,50] and imaging

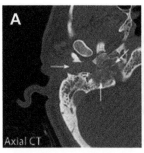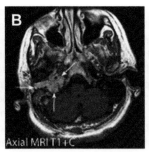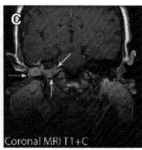

Axial CT   Axial MRI T1+C   Coronal MRI T1+C

Fig. 4. CT and MRI of a jugular paraganglioma. Jugular paragangliomas often extend to involve the hypotympanum, and show an irregular or moth-eaten appearance at the jugulo-carotid spine, jugular foramen, and/or hypoglossal canal, as seen in (*A*, *arrows*). In this particular case, the paraganglioma had extended out to the external auditory canal. On gadolinium-enhanced MRI, there is intense enhancement caused by the enormous vascularity of these tumors (*B*, axial; *C*, coronal; *arrows*). In tumors more than 2 cm, the characteristic salt-and-pepper appearance of paragangliomas corresponds to macroscopic flow voids.

is indicated before biopsy of a vascular mass in the middle ear. In addition, because paragangliomas may be multiple, contrast-enhanced CT can identify synchronous tumors of the temporal bone and upper neck.

Tympanic paragangliomas appear as well-circumscribed soft tissue masses in the middle ear, typically overlying the cochlear promontory, without gross bone erosion. Jugular paragangliomas are centered on the jugular foramen, involve the hypotympanum, and show an irregular or moth-eaten appearance of bone around their margins.[51–53] Careful attention must be given to the relationship between the tumor and the bony covering of the jugular bulb (the jugular plate). Erosion of the jugular plate suggests a jugular paraganglioma.

MRI

On MRI, paragangliomas are generally intermediate in signal on T1-weighted and T2-weighted images, enhance intensely after gadolinium administration, and larger lesions (>2 cm) show intratumoral and peritumoral flow voids that are characteristic of these tumors (the salt-and-pepper appearance) (see **Fig. 4**). MRI provides superior soft tissue details compared with HRCT because of its intrinsic soft tissue contrast resolution; additionally, because it lacks the bone artifact that is seen on CT scans,[54] it is particularly helpful to identify tumor extension intracranially. MR angiography (MRA), MRV, and catheter angiography provide information on the involvement of the great vessels and allow preoperative embolization. Compression of the internal carotid artery can be evaluated with MRA, whereas MRV can assess for occlusion of the jugular bulb and sigmoid sinus by tumor and allows assessment of collateral venous drainage.

Angiography and Embolization

Angiography serves multiple purposes. First, it provides complementary diagnostic information by showing the characteristic highly vascular nature of these lesions. However, formal intravascular angiography is not performed only for diagnostic purposes, but is combined with embolization in the preoperative period. Second, it allows identification of dominant feeding vessels that can then be embolized to reduce blood loss during surgical removal. Third, it identifies collateral vessels associated with the carotid and vertebral arteries that must be spared during surgery. Fourth, contralateral venous system patency can be fully assessed. Fifth, the presence of major venous sinus occlusion by tumor can be confirmed, and, sixth, it may help to identify multifocal tumors. Studies have shown decreased operative time and intraoperative blood loss with preoperative embolization of jugular paragangliomas,[55,56] and preoperative embolization facilitates complete resection of jugular paragangliomas. Angiography with embolization for jugular paragangliomas is usually performed 1 or 2 days before surgical excision because a longer interval between embolization and surgery may result in revascularization of the tumor, which may paradoxically increase intraoperative blood loss.[55] Because of their small size and easy accessibility, embolization of tympanic paragangliomas is not usually performed.

Nuclear Medicine Imaging

Multiple nuclear medicine–based methods have been applied for detection of head and neck paragangliomas. Octreotide is a somatostatin analogue that, when coupled to an appropriate tracer, produces a scintigraphic image of neuroendocrine tumors that express somatostatin type 2 receptors.[57] Octreotide scintigraphy imaging (the most common radioligand is ^{111}In-diethylenetriaminepentaacetic acid [DTPA]–octreotide) has been applied for the diagnosis of head and neck neuroendocrine tumors (NET) including paragangliomas, Merkel cell carcinomas, medullary thyroid carcinomas, and esthesioneuroblastomas, as well as recurrent paragangliomas (**Fig. 5**).[58,59] However, ^{111}In-DTPA-octreotide scintigraphy has limited spatial resolution and does not reliably diagnose lesions less than 1 cm.[60] Whole-body ^{123}I and ^{131}I metaiodobenzylguanidine (MIBG) scintigraphy are additional nuclear medicine

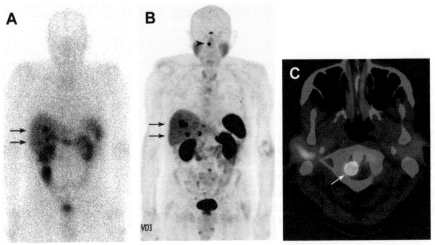

Fig. 5. Neuroendocrine tumor of the foramen magnum in an 81-year-old man with metastatic disease. (*A*) Low-resolution ^{111}In-DTPA-octreotide scintigraphy showing metastatic lesions in the liver (*black arrows*). (*B*) In the same patient as in *A*, ^{68}Ga-tetraazacyclododecane tetraacetic acid-octreotate (DOTATATE) PET/CT shows improved detail of liver metastatic disease (*black arrows*), as well as an additional metastatic lesion at the foramen magnum that was not previously seen on octreotide scintigraphy (*arrowhead*); there is physiologic uptake in the pituitary and salivary glands, spleen, and kidneys. (*C*) The foramen magnum metastasis is clearly defined on an axial PET/CT fusion (*white arrow*); there is physiologic uptake in the parotid glands.

studies that have been applied to the diagnosis of paraganglioma but also have disadvantages, including 2 patient visits because the images are captured 2 and 24 hours after tracer injection, and that the tracer accumulates in salivary glands, which may interfere with clear visualization and diagnosis.[61] MIBG whole-body scintigraphy is able to detect primary paragangliomas of the head and neck,[62] but its accuracy in detecting small paragangliomas at early stages during screening programs, especially when located in the head and neck region, is limited.[63,64] So, despite early reports of the excellent diagnostic performance of whole-body MIBG scintigraphy in the evaluation of patients with head and neck paragangliomas, this modality has not achieved a significant place in practice.[65] However, a newer generation of radiotracers has been developed, and these more specific molecular markers allow targeted molecular imaging. In addition, the use of positron-emitting radiotracers allows higher resolution images to be created that can easily be fused with CT to create high-quality maps.

NOVEL RADIOTRACERS FOR PARAGANGLIOMA IMAGING

Several novel radiotracers have been developed and tested with the goal of achieving a more comprehensive molecular fingerprint of paragangliomas of the head and neck.[59,61,66,67] In addition, a focus on positron-emitting tracers allows high-resolution clinical imaging with PET CT. Studies using ^{68}Ga-tetraazacyclododecane tetraacetic acid-Tyr-octreotide PET in NETs have shown promising results, with a higher rate of lesion identification than is achieved with conventional ^{111}In-DTPA-octreotide scintigraphy.[68–70] Another tracer, tetraazacyclododecane tetraacetic acid-octreotate (DOTATATE), is an somatostatin receptor-2 (SSTR-2) analogue that, coupled with the positron emitter ^{68}Ga, has been used for detecting NET, including paragangliomas.[60,71] In one study in patients with negative or equivocal ^{111}In-DTPA-octreotide findings, ^{68}Ga-DOTATATE PET identified additional lesions and altered management in most cases (see **Fig. 5**).[60] Another such tracer, ^{18}F-fluorodihydroxyphenylalanine (^{18}F-DOPA), is used for PET and has shown excellent results in early studies for diagnosing head and neck paragangliomas.[61] ^{18}F-DOPA is a radiolabeled dopamine precursor that is decarboxylated to dopamine inside catecholamine-secreting cells and subsequently stored in the intracellular vesicles. In one study, ^{18}F-DOPA PET showed increased accuracy in detecting paragangliomas compared with MIBG.[72] The addition of PET/CT fusions has increased specificity and sensitivity in the diagnosis of head and neck paragangliomas. One study showed that ^{18}F-DOPA PET/CT in combination was more accurate in diagnosing and localizing adrenal and extra-adrenal masses suspicious for pheochromocytomas than was ^{18}F-DOPA PET or CT alone.[73] A recent meta-analysis specifically using whole-body imaging using either ^{18}F-DOPA PET or ^{18}F-DOPA PET/CT for diagnosing paragangliomas showed 91% sensitivity and 95% specificity, although these percentages increased when patients with succinyldehydrogenase (SDHB) mutation were excluded, highlighting the importance of obtaining genetic testing.[74] Multiple studies have confirmed that ^{18}F-DOPA PET/CT performs better in detecting paragangliomas arising as part of a specific SDH syndrome. For example, the paraganglioma syndrome 1 (PGL-1–*SDHD* mutation) typically manifests as well-differentiated paragangliomas that mainly express a dopaminergic pathway and thus are ^{18}F-DOPA avid. More aggressive paragangliomas like PGL-4 (*SDHB* mutation) have reduced dopaminergic activity but have an augmented glycolytic metabolism and thus tend to have better ^{18}F-fluorodeoxyglucose (^{18}F-FDG) avidity compared with paragangliomas in the PGL-1 syndrome. Consequently, paragangliomas in patients with PGL-1 syndrome show high ^{18}F-DOPA metabolism and low ^{18}F-FDG avidity, whereas paragangliomas in PGL-4 syndrome tend to have high avidity for ^{18}F-FDG and low ^{18}F-DOPA activity.[75–77] Although CT and MR can define the presence and anatomic relationships of these lesions, molecular imaging provides an additional level of differentiation among similar-appearing tumors, and should eventually support the development of targeted therapeutics.

ARTERIAL SPIN LABELING FOR DIAGNOSING DURAL ARTERIOVENOUS FISTULAS AND ARTERIOVENOUS MALFORMATIONS

Pulsatile tinnitus is a common clinical symptom that arises from either increased blood flow or stenosis of a vascular lumen and is classified as arterial or, more commonly, as venous according to the vessel of origin.[78] The initial evaluation of a patient complaining of pulsatile tinnitus begins with a careful history and otoscopic examination. Should a middle ear mass be seen on examination, then a dedicated temporal bone CT scan should be obtained to better characterize the lesion and analyze its extent. A more difficult situation arises if the clinician does not identify any middle ear disorder. The differential diagnosis is broad, ranging from benign vascular lesions such as venous stenosis and diverticula to potentially more serious causes including DAVFs and AVMs. DAVFs and AVMs are cerebral vascular malformations characterized by arteriovenous shunting, with direct communication between the arterial and venous circulations without an intervening capillary bed. AVMs are congenital vascular malformations that most commonly affect the brain parenchyma and typically present with acute hemorrhage, seizures, or other neurologic deficits, and they uncommonly present as pulsatile tinnitus only. DAVFs are usually acquired and many causes have been proposed, including infections, trauma, surgery, venous thrombosis, neoplasms, or hypercoagulable states. DAVFs of the skull base commonly have pulsatile tinnitus alone as a presenting symptom, and the inclusion or exclusion of DAVF is often an important component of the work-up of pulsatile tinnitus.

The most common site of intracranial DAVFs is the junction of the transverse and sigmoid sinuses, and these patients often present with unilateral pulsatile tinnitus.[79] However, patients may present with more vague symptoms, such as headache. If left untreated, these lesions may have serious consequences caused by intracranial hypertension, chronic venous ischemia, and/or intracerebral hemorrhage, and hence it is crucial to diagnose these lesions and to refer them for appropriate treatment.

Digital subtraction angiography (DSA) has long been considered the gold standard for diagnosis, because its time resolution and spatial resolution allow the diagnosis of even very small DAVFs. Nevertheless, DSA is an invasive procedure that includes exposure to radiation, requires iodinated contrast injection, and carries a nonnegligible morbidity that generally relates to the risk of groin hematoma or stroke. Thus, there has been considerable interest in improving the noninvasive diagnosis of DAVF using other modalities, such as MRI/MRA/MRV (**Fig. 6**) and CT/CT angiography (CTA).[78,80,81] Narvid and colleagues[80] demonstrated the use of CTA for DAVFs. The observed CTA findings included enlarged feeding arteries, shaggy venous sinuses caused by enlarged feeder vessels, and asymmetric contrast opacification of the jugular veins; in this small study, sensitivity and specificity for DAVF exceeded 90%. MRA, either standard or time resolved, provides an additional noninvasive option for diagnosing DAVFs, but its sensitivity and specificity for small lesions are also limited. Although large DAVFs and AVMs are typically easily detected on CT/CTA or MRA/MRV, because enlarged abnormal feeding and draining vessels can be directly identified, smaller DAVFs and AVMs may present with only nonspecific imaging signs, such as secondary evidence of intracranial hypertension, and subtly enlarged vessels may be overlooked.[82]

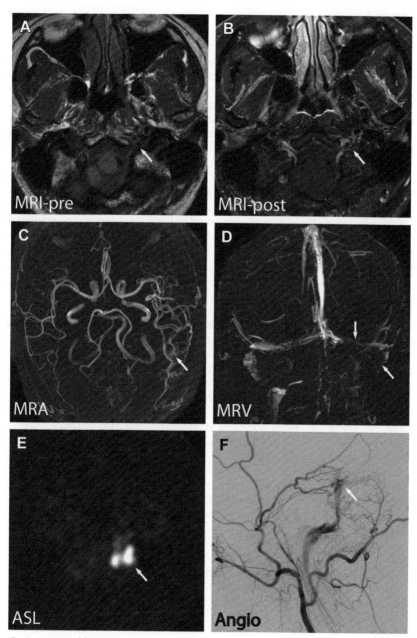

Fig. 6. A 41-year-old woman with left pulsatile tinnitus. (*A, B*) Before and after gadolinium-enhanced T1-weighted MRI (with fat saturation on *B*) showing subtle increase in vascularity with asymmetrical flow voids in the left hypoglossal canal. (*C*) MRA with asymmetrical vascularity on the left side, and subtle tangle of vessels (*arrow*). (*D*) MRV with abnormal or asymmetrical flow related enhancement in left transverse and sigmoid sinuses, signifying possible thrombosis, stenosis, or flow reversal (*arrows*). (*E*) ASL image is very low resolution, but shows intense signal down at the left skull base (*arrow*), localizing to sigmoid sinus and jugular bulb compared with other anatomic images. This finding is diagnostic of a hypervascular tumor or a shunting lesion. Because the other images show no evidence of a mass, this is consistent with an arterio-venous shunt, and the noninvasive MRI suggests a left DAVF. (*F*) Angiography, lateral view, left external carotid artery injection. Fistulous communication between multiple arterial feeders and a narrow, irregular distal transverse sinus at the transverse-sigmoid junction (*arrow*).

ASL is an emerging noncontrast, noninvasive MR technique in which arterial blood is magnetically labeled just below the region (slice) of interest by applying a 180° radio-frequency inversion pulse; using this method, the patient's own blood serves as a diffusible flow tracer downstream.[80,83] When imaging the brain under normal conditions, the labeled blood perfuses the capillary bed, and during this time it undergoes T1 decay and loses its signal.[84] However, blood that circumvents the capillary bed and is shunted directly from arteries into veins can be detected in the draining venous structures of an arteriovenous shunt lesion, because it maintains its label and hence its signal.[85] Because DAVFs and AVMs lack a capillary bed there is no water extraction and the transit time is shortened, resulting in venous ASL signal intensity (see **Fig. 6**). Le and colleagues[85] recently showed that ASL is a useful diagnostic test for DAVFs and small (<2 cm) AVMs. Although additional studies are needed, the presence or absence of venous signal on ASL should be a helpful predictor of the presence or absence of DAVF or AVM in patients with pulsatile tinnitus and no obvious vascular malformation on routine imaging studies.

REFERENCES

1. Fischbein NL, Anil K. Radiology chapter. Current diagnosis & treatment in otolaryngology head & neck surgery. 3rd edition. New York: McGraw-Hill Medical; 2011.

2. Harnsberger HR. Diagnostic imaging. Head and neck. 2nd edition. Salt Lake City (UT): Amirsys; 2011.

3. Loevner LA, Swartz JD. Imaging of the temporal bone. 4th edition. New York: Thieme; 2008.

4. Som PM, Curtin HD. Head and neck imaging. St Louis (MO): Mosby; 2011.

5. Jazrawy H, Wortzman G, Kassel EE, et al. Computed tomography of the temporal bone. J Otolaryngol 1983;12(1):37–44.

6. Mafee MF, Valvassori GE, Dobben GD. The role of radiology in surgery of the ear and skull base. Otolaryngol Clin North Am 1982;15(4):723–53.

7. Jackler RK, Dillon WP, Schindler RA. Computed tomography in suppurative ear disease: a correlation of surgical and radiographic findings. Laryngoscope 1984;94(6):746–52.

8. Lemmerling MM, De Foer B, VandeVyver V, et al. Imaging of the opacified middle ear. Eur J Radiol 2008;66(3):363–71.

9. Snow JB, Wackym PA, Ballenger JJ, ebrary Inc. Ballenger's otorhinolaryngology head and neck surgery. 17th edition. Shelton (CT); Hamilton (Canada); London: People's Medical Publishing House/BC Decker; 2009.

10. Khemani S, Singh A, Lingam RK, et al. Imaging of postoperative middle ear cholesteatoma. Clin Radiol 2011;66(8):760–7.

11. Kosling S, Bootz F. CT and MR imaging after middle ear surgery. Eur J Radiol 2001;40(2):113–8.

12. Migirov L, Tal S, Eyal A, et al. MRI, not CT, to rule out recurrent cholesteatoma and avoid unnecessary second-look mastoidectomy. Isr Med Assoc J 2009;11(3): 144–6.

13. Tierney PA, Pracy P, Blaney SP, et al. An assessment of the value of the preoperative computed tomography scans prior to otoendoscopic 'second look' in intact canal wall mastoid surgery. Clin Otolaryngol Allied Sci 1999;24(4):274–6.

14. Blaney SP, Tierney P, Oyarazabal M, et al. CT scanning in "second look" combined approach tympanoplasty. Rev Laryngol Otol Rhinol (Bord) 2000;121(2): 79–81.

15. Kashiba K, Komori M, Yanagihara N, et al. Lateral orifice of Prussak's space assessed with a high-resolution cone beam 3-dimensional computed tomography. Otol Neurotol 2011;32(1):71–6.
16. Miracle AC, Mukherji SK. Conebeam CT of the head and neck, part 1: physical principles. AJNR Am J Neuroradiol 2009;30(6):1088–95.
17. Peltonen LI, Aarnisalo AA, Kortesniemi MK, et al. Limited cone-beam computed tomography imaging of the middle ear: a comparison with multislice helical computed tomography. Acta Radiol 2007;48(2):207–12.
18. Loubele M, Bogaerts R, Van Dijck E, et al. Comparison between effective radiation dose of CBCT and MSCT scanners for dentomaxillofacial applications. Eur J Radiol 2009;71(3):461–8.
19. Berrington de Gonzalez A, Mahesh M, Kim KP, et al. Projected cancer risks from computed tomographic scans performed in the United States in 2007. Arch Intern Med 2009;169(22):2071–7.
20. Smith-Bindman R, Lipson J, Marcus R, et al. Radiation dose associated with common computed tomography examinations and the associated lifetime attributable risk of cancer. Arch Intern Med 2009;169(22):2078–86.
21. Mas-Estelles F, Mateos-Fernandez M, Carrascosa-Bisquert B, et al. Contemporary non-echo-planar diffusion-weighted imaging of middle ear cholesteatomas. Radiographics 2012;32(4):1197–213.
22. Ayache D, Williams MT, Lejeune D, et al. Usefulness of delayed postcontrast magnetic resonance imaging in the detection of residual cholesteatoma after canal wall-up tympanoplasty. Laryngoscope 2005;115(4):607–10.
23. De Foer B, Vercruysse JP, Bernaerts A, et al. Middle ear cholesteatoma: non-echo-planar diffusion-weighted MR imaging versus delayed gadolinium-enhanced T1-weighted MR imaging–value in detection. Radiology 2010;255(3):866–72.
24. Williams MT, Ayache D, Alberti C, et al. Detection of postoperative residual cholesteatoma with delayed contrast-enhanced MR imaging: initial findings. Eur Radiol 2003;13(1):169–74.
25. Hagmann P, Jonasson L, Maeder P, et al. Understanding diffusion MR imaging techniques: from scalar diffusion-weighted imaging to diffusion tensor imaging and beyond. Radiographics 2006;26(Suppl 1):S205–23.
26. Jindal M, Riskalla A, Jiang D, et al. A systematic review of diffusion-weighted magnetic resonance imaging in the assessment of postoperative cholesteatoma. Otol Neurotol 2011;32(8):1243–9.
27. Lehmann P, Saliou G, Brochart C, et al. 3T MR imaging of postoperative recurrent middle ear cholesteatomas: value of periodically rotated overlapping parallel lines with enhanced reconstruction diffusion-weighted MR imaging. AJNR Am J Neuroradiol 2009;30(2):423–7.
28. Kasbekar AV, Scoffings DJ, Kenway B, et al. Non echo planar, diffusion-weighted magnetic resonance imaging (periodically rotated overlapping parallel lines with enhanced reconstruction sequence) compared with echo planar imaging for the detection of middle-ear cholesteatoma. J Laryngol Otol 2011;125(4):376–80.
29. Khemani S, Lingam RK, Kalan A, et al. The value of non-echo planar HASTE diffusion-weighted MR imaging in the detection, localisation and prediction of extent of postoperative cholesteatoma. Clin Otolaryngol 2011;36(4):306–12.
30. Schwartz KM, Lane JI, Bolster BD Jr, et al. The utility of diffusion-weighted imaging for cholesteatoma evaluation. AJNR Am J Neuroradiol 2011;32(3):430–6.
31. Koitschev A, Behringer P, Bogner D, et al. Does diffusion-weighted MRI (DW-MRI) change treatment strategy in pediatric cholesteatoma? Acta Otolaryngol 2013; 133(5):443–8.

32. Li PM, Linos E, Gurgel RK, et al. Evaluating the utility of non-echo-planar diffusion-weighted imaging in the preoperative evaluation of cholesteatoma: a meta-analysis. Laryngoscope 2013;123(5):1247–50.

33. Majithia A, Lingam RK, Nash R, et al. Staging primary middle ear cholesteatoma with non-echoplanar (half-Fourier-acquisition single-shot turbo-spin-echo) diffusion-weighted magnetic resonance imaging helps plan surgery in 22 patients: our experience. Clin Otolaryngol 2012;37(4):325–30.

34. Profant M, Slavikova K, Kabatova Z, et al. Predictive validity of MRI in detecting and following cholesteatoma. Eur Arch Otorhinolaryngol 2012;269(3):757–65.

35. Sharifian H, Taheri E, Borghei P, et al. Diagnostic accuracy of non-echo-planar diffusion-weighted MRI versus other MRI sequences in cholesteatoma. J Med Imaging Radiat Oncol 2012;56(4):398–408.

36. Klein E. Why an MRI Costs $1,080 in America and $280 in France. The Washington Post 2012.

37. Blevins NH, Carter BL. Routine preoperative imaging in chronic ear surgery. Am J Otol 1998;19(4):527–35 [discussion: 535–8].

38. Carey JP, Minor LB, Nager GT. Dehiscence or thinning of bone overlying the superior semicircular canal in a temporal bone survey. Arch Otolaryngol Head Neck Surg 2000;126(2):137–47.

39. Fang Y, Meyer J, Chen B. High-resolution computed tomographic features of the stapedius muscle and facial nerve in chronic otitis media. Otol Neurotol 2013; 34(6):1115–20.

40. Tomlin J, Chang D, McCutcheon B, et al. Surgical technique and recurrence in cholesteatoma: a meta-analysis. Audiol Neurootol 2013;18(3):135–42.

41. Sone M, Yoshida T, Naganawa S, et al. Comparison of computed tomography and magnetic resonance imaging for evaluation of cholesteatoma with labyrinthine fistulae. Laryngoscope 2012;122(5):1121–5.

42. Wenig BM. Atlas of head and neck pathology. 2nd edition. Philadelphia: Saunders/Elsevier; 2008.

43. O'Leary MJ, Shelton C, Giddings NA, et al. Glomus tympanicum tumors: a clinical perspective. Laryngoscope 1991;101(10):1038–43.

44. Jackler RK, Brackmann DE. Neurotology. 2nd edition. Philadelphia: Elsevier Mosby; 2005.

45. Green JD Jr, Brackmann DE, Nguyen CD, et al. Surgical management of previously untreated glomus jugulare tumors. Laryngoscope 1994;104(8 Pt 1): 917–21.

46. House WF, Glasscock ME 3rd. Glomus tympanicum tumors. Arch Otolaryngol 1968;87(5):550–4.

47. Jackson CG, Welling DB, Chironis P, et al. Glomus tympanicum tumors: contemporary concepts in conservation surgery. Laryngoscope 1989;99(9):875–84.

48. Larson TC 3rd, Reese DF, Baker HL Jr, et al. Glomus tympanicum chemodectomas: radiographic and clinical characteristics. Radiology 1987;163(3):801–6.

49. Arriaga MA, Brackmann DE. Differential diagnosis of primary petrous apex lesions. Am J Otol 1991;12(6):470–4.

50. Swartz JD, Bazarnic ML, Naidich TP, et al. Aberrant internal carotid artery lying within the middle ear. High resolution CT diagnosis and differential diagnosis. Neuroradiology 1985;27(4):322–6.

51. Jackler RK, Driscoll CL. Tumors of the ear and temporal bone. Philadelphia: Lippincott Williams & Wilkins; 2000.

52. Lo WW, Solti-Bohman LG, Lambert PR. High-resolution CT in the evaluation of glomus tumors of the temporal bone. Radiology 1984;150(3):737–42.

53. Som PM, Reede DL, Bergeron RT, et al. Computed tomography of glomus tympanicum tumors. J Comput Assist Tomogr 1983;7(1):14–7.
54. Olsen WL, Dillon WP, Kelly WM, et al. MR imaging of paragangliomas. AJR Am J Roentgenol 1987;148(1):201–4.
55. Murphy TP, Brackmann DE. Effects of preoperative embolization on glomus jugulare tumors. Laryngoscope 1989;99(12):1244–7.
56. Tasar M, Yetiser S. Glomus tumors: therapeutic role of selective embolization. J Craniofac Surg 2004;15(3):497–505.
57. Telischi FF, Bustillo A, Whiteman ML, et al. Octreotide scintigraphy for the detection of paragangliomas. Otolaryngol Head Neck Surg 2000;122(3):358–62.
58. Bustillo A, Telischi F, Weed D, et al. Octreotide scintigraphy in the head and neck. Laryngoscope 2004;114(3):434–40.
59. Bustillo A, Telischi FF. Octreotide scintigraphy in the detection of recurrent paragangliomas. Otolaryngol Head Neck Surg 2004;130(4):479–82.
60. Srirajaskanthan R, Kayani I, Quigley AM, et al. The role of 68Ga-DOTATATE PET in patients with neuroendocrine tumors and negative or equivocal findings on 111In-DTPA-octreotide scintigraphy. J Nucl Med 2010;51(6):875–82.
61. Hoegerle S, Ghanem N, Altehoefer C, et al. 18F-DOPA positron emission tomography for the detection of glomus tumours. Eur J Nucl Med Mol Imaging 2003;30(5):689–94.
62. Shulkin BL, Shapiro B, Francis IR, et al. Primary extra-adrenal pheochromocytoma: positive I-123 MIBG imaging with negative I-131 MIBG imaging. Clin Nucl Med 1986;11(12):851–4.
63. Bhatia KS, Ismail MM, Sahdev A, et al. 123I-metaiodobenzylguanidine (MIBG) scintigraphy for the detection of adrenal and extra-adrenal phaeochromocytomas: CT and MRI correlation. Clin Endocrinol (Oxf) 2008;69(2):181–8.
64. Milardovic R, Corssmit EP, Stokkel M. Value of 123I-MIBG scintigraphy in paraganglioma. Neuroendocrinology 2010;91(1):94–100.
65. Ilias I, Divgi C, Pacak K. Current role of metaiodobenzylguanidine in the diagnosis of pheochromocytoma and medullary thyroid cancer. Semin Nucl Med 2011;41(5):364–8.
66. Hoegerle S, Nitzsche E, Altehoefer C, et al. Pheochromocytomas: detection with 18F DOPA whole body PET–initial results. Radiology 2002;222(2):507–12.
67. King KS, Whatley MA, Alexopoulos DK, et al. The use of functional imaging in a patient with head and neck paragangliomas. J Clin Endocrinol Metab 2010;95(2):481–2.
68. Buchmann I, Henze M, Engelbrecht S, et al. Comparison of 68Ga-DOTATOC PET and 111In-DTPAOC (Octreoscan) SPECT in patients with neuroendocrine tumours. Eur J Nucl Med Mol Imaging 2007;34(10):1617–26.
69. Gabriel M, Decristoforo C, Kendler D, et al. 68Ga-DOTA-Tyr3-octreotide PET in neuroendocrine tumors: comparison with somatostatin receptor scintigraphy and CT. J Nucl Med 2007;48(4):508–18.
70. Hofmann M, Maecke H, Borner R, et al. Biokinetics and imaging with the somatostatin receptor PET radioligand (68)Ga-DOTATOC: preliminary data. Eur J Nucl Med 2001;28(12):1751–7.
71. Kayani I, Bomanji JB, Groves A, et al. Functional imaging of neuroendocrine tumors with combined PET/CT using 68Ga-DOTATATE (DOTA-DPhe1,Tyr3-octreotate) and 18F-FDG. Cancer 2008;112(11):2447–55.
72. Fottner C, Helisch A, Anlauf M, et al. 6-18F-fluoro-L-dihydroxyphenylalanine positron emission tomography is superior to 123I-metaiodobenzyl-guanidine scintigraphy in the detection of extraadrenal and hereditary pheochromocytomas and

paragangliomas: correlation with vesicular monoamine transporter expression. J Clin Endocrinol Metab 2010;95(6):2800–10.

73. Luster M, Karges W, Zeich K, et al. Clinical value of 18F-fluorodihydroxyphenyla-lanine positron emission tomography/computed tomography (18F-DOPA PET/CT) for detecting pheochromocytoma. Eur J Nucl Med Mol Imaging 2010;37(3): 484–93.

74. Treglia G, Cocciolillo F, de Waure C, et al. Diagnostic performance of 18F-dihy-droxyphenylalanine positron emission tomography in patients with paragan-glioma: a meta-analysis. Eur J Nucl Med Mol Imaging 2012;39(7):1144–53.

75. Offergeld C, Brase C, Yaremchuk S, et al. Head and neck paragangliomas: clin-ical and molecular genetic classification. Clinics (Sao Paulo) 2012;67(Suppl 1): 19–28.

76. Rischke HC, Benz MR, Wild D, et al. Correlation of the genotype of paraganglio-mas and pheochromocytomas with their metabolic phenotype on 3,4-dihydroxy-6-18F-fluoro-L-phenylalanin PET. J Nucl Med 2012;53(9):1352–8.

77. Marzola MC, Rubello D. Molecular imaging in hereditary succinate dehydroge-nase mutation-related paragangliomas. Clin Nucl Med 2014. [Epub ahead of print].

78. Sismanis A. Pulsatile tinnitus: contemporary assessment and management. Curr Opin Otolaryngol Head Neck Surg 2011;19(5):348–57.

79. McDougall CG, Halbach VV, Dowd CF, et al. Dural arteriovenous fistulas of the marginal sinus. AJNR Am J Neuroradiol 1997;18(8):1565–72.

80. Narvid J, Do HM, Blevins NH, et al. CT angiography as a screening tool for dural arteriovenous fistula in patients with pulsatile tinnitus: feasibility and test charac-teristics. AJNR Am J Neuroradiol 2011;32(3):446–53.

81. Sismanis A. Pulsatile tinnitus. Otolaryngol Clin North Am 2003;36(2):389–402, viii.

82. Alexander M, McTaggart R, Santarelli J, et al. Multimodality evaluation of dural arteriovenous fistula with CT angiography, MR with arterial spin labeling, and dig-ital subtraction angiography: case report. J Neuroimaging 2014;24(5):520–3.

83. Alsop DC, Detre JA. Multisection cerebral blood flow MR imaging with continuous arterial spin labeling. Radiology 1998;208(2):410–6.

84. Deibler AR, Pollock JM, Kraft RA, et al. Arterial spin-labeling in routine clinical practice, part 1: technique and artifacts. AJNR Am J Neuroradiol 2008;29(7): 1228–34.

85. Le TT, Fischbein NJ, Andre JB, et al. Identification of venous signal on arterial spin labeling improves diagnosis of dural arteriovenous fistulas and small arterio-venous malformations. AJNR Am J Neuroradiol 2012;33(1):61–8.

Squamous Cell Carcinoma of the Temporal Bone

Jason A. Beyea, MD, PhD, Aaron C. Moberly, MD*

KEYWORDS

- Squamous cell carcinoma • Temporal bone malignancy • Temporal bone resection
- Cancer • External auditory canal • Surgical management

KEY POINTS

- Squamous cell carcinoma is the most common primary malignancy of the temporal bone.
- The modified University of Pittsburgh Staging System is the most commonly used system for staging temporal bone malignancies.
- Clear surgical margins improve disease-free survival.
- Postoperative radiotherapy should be offered to all patients with T2, T3, and T4 tumors.
- Multidisciplinary head and neck oncology clinics/institutional tumor boards are invaluable for optimizing the management of patients with these challenging malignancies.

CASE HISTORY

A 66-year-old man was referred to the neurotology clinic by head and neck surgery for preoperative planning. He had a 6-month history of left facial paralysis, facial numbness, otalgia, and otorrhea. Three years earlier, a left tragal squamous cell carcinoma (SCC) was resected at another institution, and he received postoperative radiation to the ear and parotid gland.

Cranial nerve examination revealed left V1 through V3 trigeminal nerve sensory deficits and a House-Brackmann grade VI/VI left facial paralysis. An extensive recurrence of the SCC was identified (**Fig. 1**). Although firmness of the left parotid was noted, no intraparotid or neck lymph nodes were palpable.

An audiogram showed pure tone averages of 5 dB on the right and 57 dB on the left. The left-sided hearing loss was a moderate sloping to profound mixed loss. A PET scan superimposed on computed tomography (CT) revealed hypermetabolic

Funding Sources: Nil.

Conflict of Interest: Nil.

Department of Otolaryngology – Head and Neck Surgery, The Ohio State University, 915 Olentangy River Road, Suite 4000, Columbus, OH 43212, USA

* Corresponding author.

E-mail address: Aaron.Moberly@osumc.edu

Abbreviations	
CRT	Chemoradiation Therapy
CT	Computed Tomography
DFS	Disease-free Survival
EAC	External Auditory Canal
LTBR	Lateral Temporal Bone Resection
SCC	Squamous Cell Carcinoma
STBR	Subtotal Temporal Bone Resection
TTBR	Total Temporal Bone Resection

activity of the left parotid gland, external auditory canal and surrounding skin, and left temporal musculature, and a small left cervical level 4/5 lymph node (**Fig. 2**). No distant metastatic disease was detected on PET. An MRI scan was performed, which revealed the presence of enhancement along the facial nerve at the left stylomastoid foramen, along V3 in the foramen ovale, and along V2 in the foramen rotundum, and enlargement of the trigeminal ganglion in Meckel's cave (**Fig. 3**). A biopsy specimen of the ear lesion revealed invasive, poorly differentiated SCC (**Fig. 4**). The patient was staged as T4N1M0; overall stage IV. His case was discussed at the authors' institutional tumor board, and the malignancy was deemed resectable. The patient decided to proceed with surgery, and informed surgical consent was obtained.

Surgery involved the head and neck oncologic surgery, neurotology, and neurosurgery teams. The resection included total auriculectomy, ipsilateral selective neck dissection (levels 2–4), parapharyngeal space tumor resection, V1/2/3 resection, temporal dura resection (**Fig. 5**), resection of involved facial nerve (with frozen section to obtain a negative proximal margin at the second genu of the nerve), lateral temporal

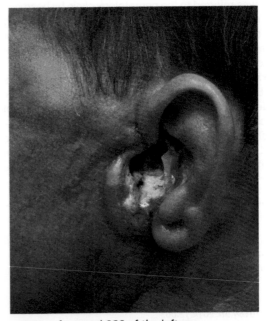

Fig. 1. Extensive recurrence of a tragal SCC of the left ear.

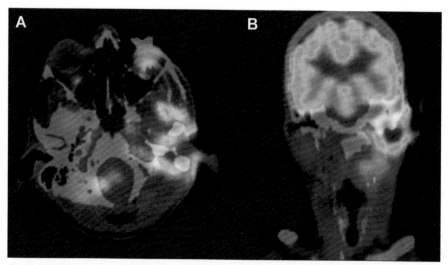

Fig. 2. PET/CT scan in axial (*A*) and coronal (*B*) sections revealed hypermetabolic activity of the left parotid gland, external auditory canal, surrounding skin, and left temporal musculature, and a small left cervical level 4/5 lymph node (lymph node not shown).

bone resection (LTBR), partial mandibulectomy (**Figs. 6** and **7**), and pectoralis major regional flap reconstruction (**Fig. 8**).

The patient's postoperative course was complicated by a cerebrospinal fluid leak at the suture line of the inferior aspect of the pectoralis flap, which was controlled by

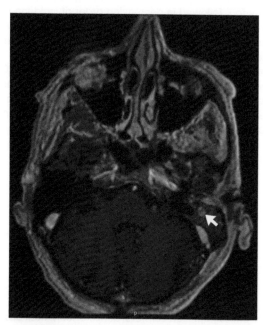

Fig. 3. Preoperative axial MRI scan (T1 with IV gadolinium). Enhancement of the distal portion of the mastoid segment of the left facial nerve is seen (*arrow*).

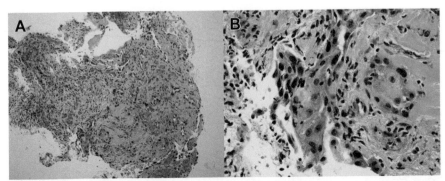

Fig. 4. Review of preoperative biopsy specimen of the tragal lesion revealed invasive poorly differentiated squamous cell carcinoma. (*A*) Low-power magnification (original magnification ×100); (*B*) high-power magnification (hematoxylin-eosin, original magnification ×400).

oversewing of the wound. He subsequently developed an infection deep to the pectoralis flap, which required intravenous antibiotics, local wound care, and finally open debridement and successful reconstruction with a myocutaneous rectus free flap. Unfortunately, on repeat MRI 3 months postoperatively, the patient developed a deep recurrence encasing the left internal carotid artery and vertebral arteries. The case was reviewed at the institutional tumor board, and the decision was made for no further intervention. The patient chose to proceed with hospice care.

PRESENTATION

Primary malignancy of the temporal bone is a rare group of neoplasms, with SCC being the most common, followed in decreasing order of incidence by basal cell carcinoma, adenocarcinoma, adenoid cystic carcinoma, mucoepidermoid carcinoma, ceruminoma, melanoma, and sarcoma.[1] Because SCC is the most common malignancy of the temporal bone, it is the focus of this publication.

The diagnosis of primary SCC of the external auditory canal (EAC) may be significantly delayed, because it is often confused with ongoing or nonresolving otitis externa. Delayed presentation often results in initial diagnosis at an advanced stage. SCC of the EAC has many possible routes of spread (**Fig. 9**), which may determine the clinical presentation.

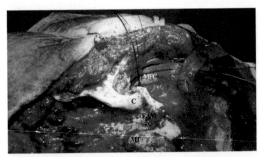

Fig. 5. Intraoperative photograph, left ear. Total auriculectomy, neck dissection, and middle fossa craniotomy have been performed. C, mandibular condyle; EAM, external auditory meatus; MFC, middle fossa craniotomy; MT, mastoid tip.

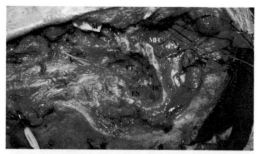

Fig. 6. Intraoperative photograph, left ear. Lateral temporal bone resection, partial mandibulectomy, facial nerve decompression, and resection to second genu of the facial nerve have been performed. ET, eustachian tube (plugged); FN, cut end of facial nerve at second genu; HC, horizontal semicircular canal; M, mandible (cut); MFC, middle fossa craniotomy.

DIAGNOSIS

A thorough history should include a search for typical symptoms, which, in decreasing order of frequency, include otalgia, otorrhea, decreased hearing, facial palsy, and parotid mass.[2] The risk factors are chronic irritation or inflammation,[3] in sharp contrast to the typical risk factors for cutaneous SCC on sun-exposed regions of the body. Comprehensive examination of the head and neck includes evaluation of the extent of the primary lesion, cranial nerve examination, and palpation of the parotid gland and neck in search of lymphadenopathy. An audiogram is obtained, both to evaluate the extent and type of hearing loss in the affected ear and to evaluate the contralateral hearing, which is vital should extensive surgical intervention be planned.

Imaging

High-resolution CT of the temporal bone is the standard for assessing bone erosion as a result of malignancy.[4] Preoperative CT is able to detect all bone erosions of 2 mm or greater.[5] MRI is complementary, because it provides detailed soft tissue resolution, distinction between tumor and fluid, assessment for intracranial involvement,

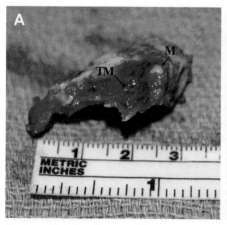
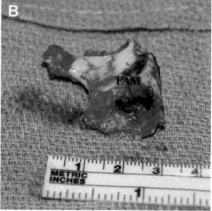

Fig. 7. Lateral temporal bone specimen: (A) medial aspect, (B) lateral aspect. EAM, external auditory meatus; M, malleus (head); TM, tympanic membrane.

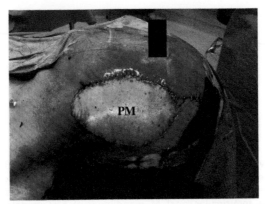

Fig. 8. Postoperative photograph, left ear. Reconstruction has been performed with a pectoralis major flap (PM).

identification of perineural spread, and evaluation of the major blood vessels of the skull base.

Biopsy

Definitive diagnosis is achieved through biopsy of the primary lesion, which is typically performed under local anesthetic (see **Fig. 4**).

Metastatic Workup

CT scan with intravenous contrast of the neck will reveal regional lymph nodes. Evaluation for distal metastases is most often performed with a chest CT with intravenous

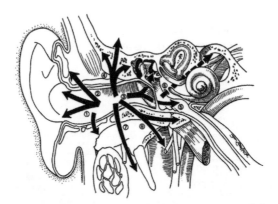

Fig. 9. Coronal anatomy of pathways of spread of primary cancer of the external auditory canal. Cancer can spread (1) anteriorly through the cartilaginous canal into the parotid gland, (2) through the concha into the postauricular sulcus, (3) through the tympanic membrane into the middle ear, (4) posteriorly into the mastoid, (5) into the anterior mesotympanum to the carotid artery and eustachian tube, (6) into the inner ear through the round window or otic capsule, (7) along the extratemporal facial nerve into the infratemporal fossa, and (8) inferomedially into the jugular fossa, carotid artery, and lower cranial nerves. (*From* Moody SA, Hirsch BE, Myers EN. Squamous cell carcinoma of the external auditory canal: an evaluation of a staging system. Am J Otol 2000;21:582–8; with permission.)

contrast, or a chest radiograph. Alternatively, a PET scan from the skull base to the lower extremities can be used to identify hypermetabolic loci suggestive of metastatic carcinoma.

STAGING

A universally accepted staging system for temporal bone carcinoma currently does not exist. However, the most widely used staging for SCC of the temporal bone is the modified University of Pittsburgh Staging System (**Table 1**).[6] This system highlights the grim prognosis for patients with lymph node involvement and/or distant metastases.

TREATMENT

Although consensus is lacking regarding the management of SCC of the temporal bone, a general treatment strategy is presented in **Table 2**.[7,8] **Fig. 10** demonstrates the surgical margins and structures involved in various temporal bone resection approaches.

Table 1
Modified University of Pittsburgh Staging System for SCC of the temporal bone

Status	Description
T status	
T1	Tumor limited to the external auditory canal without bony erosion or evidence of soft tissue extension
T2	Tumor with limited external auditory canal bony erosion (not full thickness) or radiographic finding consistent with limited (<0.5 cm) soft tissue involvement
T3	Tumor eroding the osseous external auditory canal (full thickness) with limited (<0.5 cm) soft tissue involvement, or tumor involving middle ear and/or mastoid
T4	Tumor eroding the cochlea, petrous apex, medial wall of the middle ear, carotid canal, jugular foramen, or dura, or with extensive (>0.5 cm) soft tissue involvement; patients presenting with facial paralysis
N status	
N0	No regional nodes identified
N1	Single ipsilateral regional node <3 cm
N2a	Single ipsilateral regional node 3–6 cm
N2b	Multiple ipsilateral regional nodes ≤6 cm
N2c	Bilateral or contralateral regional nodes ≤6 cm
N3	Regional node >6 cm
M status	
M0	Absence of distant metastatic disease
M1	Presence of distant metastatic disease
Overall stage	
I	T1N0M0
II	T2N0M0
III	T3N0M0
IV	T4N0M0, T1–4N+M0, T1–4N0–3M1

Data from Refs.[1,6]

Table 2
Treatment of SCC of the temporal bone based on stage

Stage	Treatment
T1	LTBR or primary radiation, consider SP
T2	LTBR plus postoperative radiation, consider SP
T3	STBR or TTBR plus postoperative radiation, consider SP
T4	STBR or TTBR plus postoperative radiation, consider SP
N+	Add radical parotidectomy and SND to the above
M+	Palliation

Abbreviations: LTBR, lateral temporal bone resection; SND, selective neck dissection; SP, superficial parotidectomy; STBR, subtotal temporal bone resection; TTBR, total temporal bone resection.
  Data from Refs.[7,8]

En Bloc Versus Piecemeal Removal

Types of resections of malignancies of the temporal bone include sleeve resection, LTBR, subtotal temporal bone resection (STBR), and total temporal bone resection (TTBR). Because temporal bone resections involve significant tissue loss and exposure of vital structures, reconstruction with vascularized tissue is of paramount importance. Careful preoperative planning with a head and neck reconstructive surgeon will help achieve the optimal postoperative outcome.

Sleeve resection involves the removal of the cartilaginous portion of the EAC, the skin of the bony EAC, and possibly the tympanic membrane, leaving the bony EAC intact. This procedure should only be considered for low-grade lesions of the EAC skin that do not involve bone. SCC of the EAC requires, at a minimum, an LTBR.

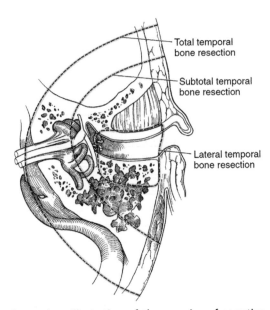

Fig. 10. Margins of resection. Illustration of the margins of resection based on type of temporal bone resection. (*From* Marsh M, Jenkins HA. Temporal bone neoplasms and lateral cranial base surgery. In: Flint PW, Haughey BH, Lund V, editors. Cummings Otolaryngology - Head and Neck Surgery, 5th edition. New York: Elsevier; 2010. p. 2492; with permission.)

LTBR involves removal of the cartilaginous and bony EAC, tympanic membrane, malleus, and incus. This technique is typically performed in an en bloc fashion through an extended facial recess approach with sacrifice of the chorda tympani. The facial nerve and inner ear are entirely preserved.

STBR is indicated when malignancy has extended to the middle ear. This surgery involves starting with an en bloc LTBR. Further dissection is dictated by the extent of tumor spread. If involved, the facial nerve is resected to the extent needed to obtain a negative frozen section, and consideration is given to facial nerve grafting. Drilling continues medially into the otic capsule and petrous temporal bone until negative margins are obtained. The internal carotid artery is preserved.

TTBR includes the resection margins of an STBR, but also involves resection of the petrous apex, sigmoid sinus, and possibly the petrous segment of the internal carotid artery. Internal carotid artery resection should only be considered after preoperative assessment of cerebral blood flow. This technique typically includes 30-minute temporary balloon occlusion of the internal carotid artery. Patients who display neurologic deficits during this occlusion are considered to be at high risk for stroke if the carotid is resected. A more conservative surgical resection should be considered for these patients. TTBR has a risk of significantly higher morbidity compared with STBR, and a survival benefit has yet to be proven. Pragmatic discussion of risks and benefits with the patient, combined with a multidisciplinary discussion of the case at the institutional tumor board, will guide appropriate therapy.

The goal of surgical treatment is to remove all malignancy while minimizing damage to or sacrifice of vital structures. The debate regarding whether patients are optimally treated with en bloc versus piecemeal resection has not been resolved. En bloc removal of the EAC is typically straightforward. Resection of disease medial to the EAC can be performed with less intraoperative risk using a piecemeal approach. If performing piecemeal resection, frozen sections will guide successful extirpation of disease.

Role of Parotidectomy and Neck Dissection

Therapeutic parotidectomy and neck dissection are performed if these structures contain local and/or lymphatic spread of disease. Preoperative imaging is essential in the evaluation of local/regional spread. The role of prophylactic parotidectomy with or without neck dissection is more controversial. **Table 2** presents a useful treatment algorithm. Generally, prophylactic parotidectomy with or without neck dissection is considered in patients with advanced T-stage disease (T3 or T4). Mazzoni and colleagues[9] reviewed their series of 41 consecutive patients with SCC of the EAC. They advocated total parotidectomy for anterior growth beyond the anterior wall of the EAC, and a prophylactic superficial parotidectomy in T1 and T2 cases. A modified radical neck dissection was performed for clinically positive lymph nodes, and a prophylactic selective neck dissection was performed in patients with clinically negative necks who underwent LTBR or STBR. Neck dissection was not performed in some elderly patients with N0 necks, or in patients with advanced tumor with poor prognosis.

The approach of Mazzoni and colleagues[9] favored more aggressive use of prophylactic parotidectomy/neck dissection than that used by other authors.[7,8] The rarity of these tumors makes the role of prophylactic parotidectomy and neck dissection difficult to study. Future publications that stratify prognosis based on whether these procedures were performed will help guide clinical decision making.

Role of Adjuvant Therapies

Postoperative radiotherapy using a dose of 50 to 60 Gy is typically offered to all patients with T2, T3, or T4 disease who are well enough to tolerate radiation.[10] Consultation with a radiation oncologist will guide decisions regarding chemotherapy.

Currently, the role of chemotherapy is undefined. In general, chemotherapy should be considered for patients with T4 tumors, residual disease after surgery, or metastatic disease.[11] Cisplatin is the preferred chemotherapeutic agent. Of particular interest, Takenaka and colleagues[8] performed a meta-analysis of patients with SCC of the EAC, and found an improved overall 5-year survival rate of 85.7% in patients treated with preoperative chemoradiation (CRT) followed by surgery, compared with surgery with or without radiation (53.5%), definitive CRT (43.6%), and postoperative CRT (0%). Although the subgroup treated with preoperative CRT consisted of a small number of patients, this promising potential treatment requires further evaluation. Consultation with a medical oncologist will guide decisions surrounding the use of chemotherapy.

Indications for Palliative Therapy

In patients with N+ disease, involvement of the carotid artery, or poorly differentiated SCC on histology, palliative therapy should be considered.[10] Masterson and colleagues[10] found that dural or brain invasion did not negatively affect survival. However, Moody and colleagues[2] found that 0% of their patients with dural invasion were alive 2 years later, compared with 56% of those whose dura was not involved (or not explored). Taken together, these findings suggest that tumors with dural or brain involvement may be amenable to surgical resection. Multidisciplinary oncologic medical teams are extremely valuable in determining the overall treatment direction of patients with SCC of the temporal bone.

Management of the Facial Nerve

If preoperative clinical facial weakness exists, resection of the nerve is performed until a negative margin is achieved.[12] In patients with normal facial function, tumor adherence to bone of the stylomastoid foramen is also an indication for nerve resection. Furthermore, tumor adherence to the nerve at other locations may necessitate nerve resection. If resected, nerve grafting is considered. Donor tissue options include the great auricular nerve, sural nerve, or lateral antebrachial cutaneous nerve.

Importance of Surgical Margins

The oncologic goal for surgery of the temporal bone for SCC is to obtain clear margins. Essig and colleagues[13] found that a clear margin was associated with disease-free survival (DFS) rate of 81% at 2 years, in contrast to a DFS rate of 45% in patients with a positive margin. Moody and colleagues[2] similarly found that positive histologic margins were associated with a decreased survival rate at 2 years (32%) compared with clear margins (75%).

PROGNOSIS

The 2-year survival rates reported for patients who have undergone surgical resection with or without adjuvant radiotherapy vary considerably by study. Prasad and colleagues[4] reviewed the literature and reported ranges of survival for T1 (48%–100%), T2 (28%–100%), T3 (17%–100%), and T4 (14.3%–54.0%) tumors. These discrepancies in survival illustrate the difficulty in studying these rare malignancies. In addition to a lower T stage, other positive prognostic factors previously discussed include absence of nodal or distant metastases, and clear surgical margins. The prognostic role of en bloc versus piecemeal resection currently has not been resolved.

Conversely, negative prognostic factors include advanced T stage, N+ disease, M+ disease, and positive surgical margins.

SUMMARY

SCC of the temporal bone is a challenging clinical entity. A thorough workup includes history, physical examination, biopsy, appropriate imaging, and a metastatic workup. The modified University of Pittsburgh Staging System is used for staging. The authors recommend discussion of these cases at multidisciplinary head and neck oncology clinics/institutional tumor boards to optimize treatment outcomes. The scope of surgery depends on the extent of tumor and involvement of critical structures. Postoperative radiotherapy should be offered to patients with T2, T3, and T4 tumors. Consultation with a medical oncologist will help determine whether additional benefit can be obtained from chemotherapy.

ACKNOWLEDGMENT

The authors would like to thank Dr Alejandro A. Gru (Department of Pathology, The Ohio State University) for providing the pathology images used in **Fig. 4**.

REFERENCES

1. Bacciu A, Clemente IA, Piccirillo E, et al. Guidelines for treating temporal bone carcinoma based on long-term outcomes. Otol Neurotol 2013;34:898–907.
2. Moody SA, Hirsch BE, Myers EN. Squamous cell carcinoma of the external auditory canal: an evaluation of a staging system. Am J Otol 2000;21:582–8.
3. Gaudet JE, Walvekar RR, Arriaga MA, et al. Applicability of the Pittsburgh staging system for advanced cutaneous malignancy of the temporal bone. Skull Base 2010;20:409–14.
4. Prasad SC, D'Orazio F, Medina M, et al. State of the art in temporal bone malignancies. Curr Opin Otolaryngol Head Neck Surg 2014;22:154–65.
5. Hosokawa S, Mizuta K, Takahashi G, et al. Surgical approach for treatment of carcinoma of the anterior wall of the external auditory canal. Otol Neurotol 2012;33: 450–4.
6. Hirsch BE. Staging system revision. Arch Otolaryngol Head Neck Surg 2002;128: 93–4.
7. Leong SC, Youssef A, Lesser TH. Squamous cell carcinoma of the temporal bone: outcomes of radical surgery and postoperative radiotherapy. Laryngoscope 2013;123:2442–8.
8. Takenaka Y, Cho H, Nakahara S, et al. Chemoradiation therapy for squamous cell carcinoma of the external auditory canal: a meta-analysis. Head Neck 2014. [Epub ahead of print].
9. Mazzoni A, Danesi G, Zanoletti E. Primary squamous cell carcinoma of the external auditory canal: surgical treatment and long-term outcomes. Acta Otorhinolaryngol Ital 2014;34:129–37.
10. Masterson L, Rouhani M, Donnelly NP, et al. Squamous cell carcinoma of the temporal bone: clinical outcomes from radical surgery and postoperative radiotherapy. Otol Neurotol 2014;35:501–8.
11. Kunst H, Lavieille JP, Marres H. Squamous cell carcinoma of the temporal bone: results and management. Otol Neurotol 2008;29:549–52.

12. Shao A, Wong DK, McIvor NP, et al. Parotid metastatic disease from cutaneous squamous cell carcinoma: prognostic role of facial nerve sacrifice, lateral temporal bone resection, immune status and P-stage. Head Neck 2014;36:545–50.
13. Essig GF, Kitipornchai L, Adams F, et al. Lateral temporal bone resection in advanced cutaneous squamous cell carcinoma: report of 35 patients. J Neurol Surg B Skull Base 2013;74:54–9.

Glomus Tympanicum Tumors

Alex D. Sweeney, MD[a],*, Matthew L. Carlson, MD[b], George B. Wanna, MD[a], Marc L. Bennett, MD[a]

KEYWORDS

- Glomus tympanicum • Tympanic paraganglioma • Middle ear tumor

KEY POINTS

- Glomus tympanicum (GT) arise from paraganglion cells of the middle ear and are distinguished from glomus jugulare by a lack of bony erosion around the jugular bulb.
- At a minimum, all patients with a suspected GT should have a high-resolution computed tomography of the temporal bone and neck for diagnostic purposes.
- Genetic testing and evaluation for tumor neurosecretory function should be considered based on a patient's history and demographic information.
- Surgical resection is the best option for definitive treatment of GT tumors.
- During surgical resection, avoid unnecessary morbidity by leaving adherent disease on vital structures when necessary.

 Videos of the pulsation of a temporal bone paraganglioma behind an intact tympanic membrane and stepwise, microsurgical resection of an anteriorly based glomus tympanicum accompany this article at http://www.oto.theclinics.com/

INTRODUCTION

Glomus tympanicum (GT) tumors, or tympanic paraganglioma, are the most common benign tumors of the middle ear.[1] Paragangliomas are embryologically derived from the neural crest and represent a proliferation of paraganglion cells within a highly vascular environment. These cells are normally associated with structures of the autonomic nervous system throughout the body and are most abundant in the adrenal

Financial Material & Support: Internal departmental funding was used without commercial sponsorship or support.
Conflict(s) of Interest to Declare: There are no relevant disclosures.
[a] Department of Otolaryngology-Head and Neck Surgery, Vanderbilt University, Nashville, TN 37232, USA; [b] Department of Otolaryngology-Head and Neck Surgery, Mayo Clinic School of Medicine, Rochester, MN 55905, USA
* Corresponding author. Department of Otolaryngology-Head and Neck Surgery, The Bill Wilkerson Center for Otolaryngology & Communication Sciences, 7209 Medical Center East, South Tower 1215, 21st Avenue South, Nashville, TN 37232-8605.
E-mail address: alex.d.sweeney@vanderbilt.edu

glands. Neoplastic proliferations of paraganglion cells arising from the adrenal glands are called *pheochromocytomas*, whereas extra-adrenal paragangliomas are most frequently found in the head and neck and have been referred to as *chemodectomas* and *glomus tumors*.[2]

Paragangliomas of the head and neck are most commonly found at the carotid body and represent less than 1% of tumors in this region.[3] Within the temporal bone, para-ganglioma tumors arise along the tympanic plexus of the Arnold and Jacobson nerves or the adventitia of the jugular bulb.[4] The former are called *tympanic paraganglioma*, and the latter are called *jugular paraganglioma*. These tumors are also referred to as *glomus tympanicum* and *glomus jugulare*, respectively.

Although surgical resection of tympanic paragangliomas continues to be the best option for definitive treatment, the diagnostic and management algorithms for these lesions have evolved over time. Tumor diagnosis begins clinically with the visualiza-tion of a red mass behind an intact eardrum, but computed tomography (CT) and MRI have become essential for identifying the tumor origin and defining the extent of disease. Screening for tumors with neuroendocrine secretory function remains of critical importance in select cases, and with the increasing sophistication and avail-ability of genetic testing, the implications of patient specific tumor biology are an emerging consideration. From a surgical perspective, the generally benign nature of these tumors juxtaposed with their close proximity to the facial nerve, cochleo-vestibular system, jugular vein, and internal carotid artery have led to recommenda-tions for less aggressive resection to avoid unnecessary morbidity in the setting of adherent disease. This article provides an in depth discussion of GT pathophysi-ology and a review of historical and contemporary trends in tumor diagnosis and management.

HISTORY

Paraganglioma of the temporal bone emerged as a distinct pathologic entity during the 20th century. Stacy R. Guild[5] first described the existence of naturally occurring glomus formations along the Jacobson and Arnold nerves in the 1940s. Rose-nwasser[6] subsequently explained paraganglioma growth as a neoplastic proliferation of these structures, and Simpson and Dallachy[7] reviewed reported cases of vascular middle ear tumors dating as far back as 1889, concluding that many were likely to have been paragangliomas. Using this work, Guild[8] was able to perform a general analysis of tumor anatomy in which he noted that the vascular pedicle for most tu-mors was the ascending pharyngeal artery. However, many subsequent tumor char-acterizations were hindered by difficulty distinguishing GT from jugulare. In a 1962 meta-analysis of 316 tumors, Alford and Guilford[9] noted that a "multiplicity of loca-tion from which these tumors may arise" complicates a description of "definite symp-toms or symptom complexes that will satisfy all these tumors and/or be pathognomonic of all of them." However, this confusion did not prevent the identifi-cation of important demographic and symptom trends associated with temporal bone paragangliomas. Alford and Guilford[9] found that affected patients were more commonly women (66%) and middle-aged (mean, 49 years; range, 17–85 years). Patients were most likely to present with hearing loss, tinnitus, and a red, bulging tympanic membrane or a polypoid mass in the external auditory canal (EAC). Less than 5% of patients had multifocal tumors, with even fewer experiencing metastatic or secretory disease.[9]

Complete surgical resection has historically been the preferred treatment for GT. House and Glasscock[10] described the importance of preoperative polytomography and retrograde jugulography for accurate diagnosis, and standardized surgical approaches as either transcanal or postauricular depending on the presumed tumor extent. For cases in which the tumor was locally advanced, a postauricular incision allowed for a mastoidectomy, posterior tympanotomy, extended facial recess, and fallopian bridge. The importance of functional preservation was also reinforced with the recommendation that "the posterior canal wall, the tympanic membrane, ossicles, and facial nerve should remain intact".[10] The collective experience of these authors set the general standards for GT surgery that persist into the current era of operative management.

TUMOR HISTOLOGY AND PATHOPHYSIOLOGY

A histologic analysis of GT tumors reveals many similarities to paragangliomas that occur elsewhere in the body. Grossly, tumors are solid and encapsulated, although they can often have an invasive appearance in the temporal bone because of growth within haversian canals and air cells.[2] Microscopically, tumors are conglomerations of chief cells surrounded by sustentacular cells ("zellballen") and an extensive capillary network that creates a reticular appearance (**Fig. 1**). Chief cells are characterized by a polyhedral shape, round nuclei, and eosinophilic cytoplasm that can contain granular structures (**Fig. 2**).[11] Immunohistochemical staining generally reveals chromogranin, serotonin, neuron-specific enolase, and somatostatin expression in chief cells and S-100 expression in sustentacular cells.

Neurosecretory function in GT tumors is rare, but screening for functional tumors remains an important part of tumor management. Pheochromocytomas of the adrenal medulla are not uncommonly secretory and are able to produce dopamine,

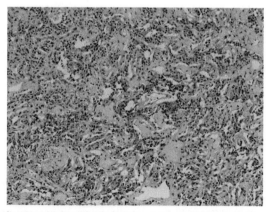

Fig. 1. Low-magnification histopathology of a temporal bone paraganglioma. The Zellballen architecture is visible, along with a richly vascular stroma and focal fibrosis (Hematoxylin and Eosin stain).

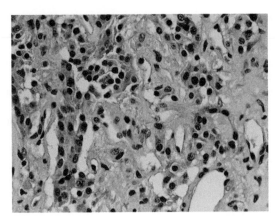

Fig. 2. High-magnification histopathology of a temporal bone paraganglioma. The chief cells are small with basophilic cytoplasm and have round, granular nuclei (Hematoxylin and Eosin stain).

norepinephrine, and epinephrine. However, functional head and neck tumors are only seen in 1% to 3% of cases[2,12,13] and, because of a lack of the enzyme phenyl-ethanolamine-*N*-methyltransferase, which is not commonly found in extramedullary paragangliomas, norepinephrine secretion predominates.[14,15] Although the incidence of neurosecretory function in GT tumors is low, the autonomic instability provoked by catecholamine release during surgical manipulation necessitates careful screening during tumor workup. Historically, preoperative venous sampling was encouraged in all cases to avoid a rare intraoperative crisis.[16,17] Presently, the identification of functional tumors relies on a preoperative workup that includes a detailed medical history and laboratory testing designed to identify an excess of catecholamines or their byproducts in the systemic circulation or urine. The details of this workup are discussed in more detail later.

Despite being prone to locally aggressive behavior, GT tumors are generally benign histologically. According to multiple sources, malignancy is ultimately identified in approximately 5% of temporal bone paragangliomas.[18–20] Although some have suggested that microscopic evidence of increased mitotic activity, necrosis, and local invasion can be indicators of malignancy, a histopathologic basis currently does not exist for distinguishing between benign and malignant disease. Rather, the presence of regional or distant metastasis serves as the most widely accepted trait of malignancy.[21,22]

The genetic basis of paraganglioma development is an emerging topic. Ten percent of head and neck paraganglioma are believed to be familial in nature,[23] and previous work has identified multiple potential loci on chromosome 11, termed *paraganglioma loci* (PGL), that seem to play a role in tumor pathogenesis.[24–26] Inheritance via an autosomal dominant pattern influenced by genomic imprinting has been described.[27] Subsequent studies have revealed mutations in succinate dehydrogenase (SDH) complexes at these locations that are believed to be responsible for familial tumor pathogenesis.[28] Because the phenotypes associated with distinct mutations may differ,[29,30] the genetic origin of a glomus tumor may also have implications on its malignant potential, particularly in the case of SDHB mutations.[31]

PRESENTATION: DEMOGRAPHICS AND CLINICAL EVALUATION

GT tumors are more commonly seen in specific patient populations. A strong female predilection was reported previously,[32,33] and this trend was verified by a recent review of the authors' experience at The Otology Group of Vanderbilt, in which 90.4% of patients were women, the mean age at presentation was 55.2 years (range, 25.9–79.1 years), and bimodal peaks were seen in patients in their 30s and 60s.[34] The authors also observed that men with GT typically present at a younger age. In other reports, tumors have even been diagnosed in infants.[35] A significant preponderance in tumor laterality was not seen (52.2% right-sided), which is consistent with what has been previously described.[33]

The history and physical examination are an important part of the evaluation of a patient with a suspected GT. Patients commonly present with complaints of pulsatile tinnitus (81.4%), subjective hearing loss (77.1%), and aural fullness (70.2%), whereas otalgia is uncommon.[34] In extensive tumors that have grown though the tympanic membrane, episodic bloody otorrhea can occur (9.6%).[34] Rarely, growth within the eustachian tube can lead to epistaxis.[36] Symptoms suggestive of lower cranial neuropathy, such as dysphonia, dysphagia, and weakness of the shoulder or tongue, should raise suspicion for a jugular paraganglioma. Preoperative facial paralysis was seen in only one patient in the authors' series (0.9%), who presented 9 years after a subtotal resection at an outside center.[34] On otoscopic examination, tumors are generally recognizable as red, pulsatile masses of the middle ear (**Fig. 3**, Video 1). When the mass is in contact with the tympanic membrane, blanching can occasionally be seen with pneumatic pressure, which is referred to as Brown's sign. In the authors' series, Brown's sign was documented in approximately half of the cases.[34] In additional to a history and physical examination, baseline audiometry should always be performed during the initial evaluation to objectively evaluate the degree to which a tumor has affected hearing.

DIAGNOSTIC IMAGING AND STAGING

Diagnostic imaging is essential to the workup of a suspected tympanic paraganglioma to exclude other possible diagnoses and define the extent of disease.

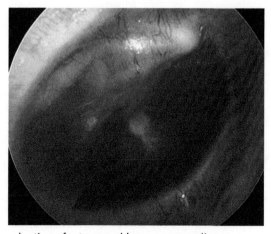

Fig. 3. Otoscopic evaluation of a temporal bone paraganglioma.

The presence of a red, pulsatile mass in the middle ear is not an exclusive feature of a paraganglioma,[37] and even among the 2 forms of temporal bone paraganglioma, the clinical presentation can be essentially identical.[38–40] High-resolution CT remains the preferred diagnostic modality to visualize the relationship of a suspected tumor to surrounding bone. Erosion around the jugular bulb is considered to be characteristic of a jugular paraganglioma, which arises from paraganglion cells in the venous adventitia (**Fig. 4**). MRI, with and without contrast, is generally preferred to CT when evaluating the soft tissue component of a tumor. The characteristic appearance of a paraganglioma on contrast-enhanced MRI is the so-called salt-and-pepper pattern most evident on T2-weighted sequences, representing prominent intratumoral flow voids. Although tumors confined to the middle ear may not require MRI evaluation to visualize tumor extent, the added value of an MRI in the setting of a locally advanced GT may help distinguish the tumor from trapped secretions in the temporal bone. Although conventional angiography has been used in the past to evaluate for synchronous lesions in the head and neck, CT and MRI have replaced this modality in the authors' practice. Our preference is to, at a minimum, perform high-resolution CT of the temporal bone and neck with and without contrast when evaluating a new patient with a GT. MRI or magnetic resonance angiography can be performed as an adjunct to CT when additional clarification regarding adjacent soft tissue is required.

Tumor staging is an important element of the diagnostic algorithm for GT tumors. Two separate staging systems are commonly referenced: Fisch-Mattox[41] and Glasscock-Jackson.[1] The Fisch-Mattox system incorporates both tympanic and jugular paraganglioma into one continuum (**Table 1**), although Sanna and colleagues[33] proposed a modified version that is specific to tympanicum tumors (**Table 2**). The Glasscock-Jackson staging system separates tympanic and jugular tumors, and the tympanic classification is listed in **Table 3**.

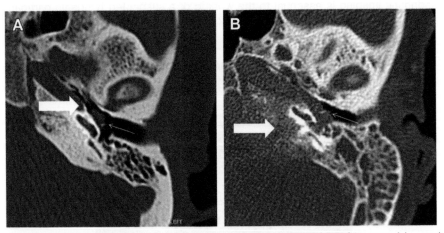

Fig. 4. CT evaluation of temporal bone paraganglioma. (*A*) GT (*thin white arrow*) located anteriorly in the middle ear cavity. The bone of the carotid canal is intact over the carotid artery (*thick white arrow*). (*B*) Glomus jugulare (*thin white arrow*) arising from the jugular foramen, causing bony erosion (*thick white arrow*) to distinguish it from a GT.

Table 1
The Fisch-Mattox classification system

Grade	Definition
A	Tumor entirely within the middle ear space
B	Tumor only within the middle ear or mastoid portion of the temporal bone
C	Tumor within the infralabyrinthine temporal bone or petrous apex
D1	Tumors with <2 cm of intracranial extension
D2	Tumors with ≥2 cm of intracranial extension

From Fisch U. Infratemporal fossa approach for extensive tumors of the temporal bone and base of skull. In: Silverstein H, Norrell H, editors. Neurological surgery of the ear. Birmingham (AL): Aesculapius; 1977. p. 34–53.

ADDITIONAL WORKUP

Laboratory evaluation can be a helpful adjunct when diagnosing GT tumors, particularly when concern exists for a secreting tumor. As previously mentioned, a balance must be struck between the consequences of unexpected catecholamine release during tumor dissection and superfluous laboratory testing, given the rarity of neurosecretory function. Previous literature has supported the use of urine and plasma screening for catecholamines and their metabolites (metanephrine, normetanephrine, and vanillylmandelic acid) in all patients with a GT tumor.[40] The authors' approach generally involves investigation for a secretory tumor in cases of familial disease, multifocal disease, or when suggestive symptoms are elicited in the history, such as diarrhea, headaches, flushing, hypertension, and palpations.

The utility of genetic screening in the contemporary management of GT tumors is becoming increasingly apparent. Specific mutation analysis has been shown to have predictive value for neurosecretory function,[42] malignant transformation,[31] and synchronous disease burden. Recent evidence indicates that elective screening would be a valuable adjunct for patients younger than 40 years, with multicentric disease, or with a family history of paraganglioma tumors.[43] When familial inheritance is suspected, a stepwise progression of locus testing, beginning with SDHD and SDHB, is considered a cost-effective approach.[44]

TREATMENT

Surgery remains the only viable option for definitive tumor management.[40] When considering resection, preoperative treatment planning is essential, particularly for

Table 2
The modified Fisch-Mattox classification system

Grade	Definition
A1	Tumor margins completely visible on otoscopy
A2	Tumor margins not completely visible on otoscopy
B1	Tumor filling the middle ear and extending into the hypotympanum or sinus tympani
B2	Tumor filling the middle ear and in the mastoid
B3	Tumor eroding into the carotid canal

From Sanna M, Fois P, Pasanisi E, et al. Middle ear and mastoid glomus tumors (glomus tympanicum): an algorithm for the surgical management. Auris Nasus Larynx 2010;37(6):661–8.

Table 3	
The Glasscock-Jackson classification system	
Grade	**Definition**
1	Tumor margins completely visible on otoscopy
2	Tumor filling the middle ear
3	Tumor filling the middle ear and in the mastoid
4	Tumor extending through the tympanic membrane into the external auditory canal

From Jackson CG, Leonetti JP, Marz SJ. Surgery for benign tumors of the temporal bone. Glasscock-Shambaugh surgery of the ear. 6th edition. In: Gulya AJ, Minor LB, Poe DS, editors. Shelton (CT): People's Medical Publishing House; 2010. p. 729–50.

managing intraoperative blood loss and the possible need for pharmacologic intervention. If a tumor is found to have neurosecretory function, the expertise of an endocrinologist should be sought to help determine whether perioperative α-adrenergic and possibly β-adrenergic blockades are necessary. Particular care should be taken with patients who use a β-blocker drug for hypertension control, because these individuals are at risk for an overwhelming α-agonist response with catecholamine release.[45] Embolization is generally not recommended for tympanicum tumors.

The surgical approach to a GT can usually be predicted by the stage of the tumor. For Glasscock-Jackson class 1 lesions, in which the tumor margins can be seen during otoscopy, transcanal excision is generally achievable. Otherwise, a postauricular incision should be planned. A simple mastoidectomy is helpful to visualize tumors that extend superiorly into the attic. An extended posterior tympanotomy or hypotympanotomy can be performed to access tumors that extend inferiorly.[40,46] For advanced tumors that have eroded through the bony EAC, modified radical mastoidectomy, with or without canal overclosure, can be necessary. In the authors' experience, the paradigm for surgical approaches has been stable during the past 40 years. Transcanal excisions are performed for most cases of Glasscock-Jackson class 1 disease, and tympanomastoidectomy with either facial recess or hypotympanotomy is used for most Glasscock-Jackson class 2 and 3 disease, with a trend toward using the latter in more recent years. For Glasscock-Jackson class 4 disease, canal wall down mastoidectomy with meatoplasty or ear canal overclosure is performed if a large canal defect is present.[34]

Tympanic paraganglioma resection can be a complicated endeavor given the vascular nature of the tumor and the proximity of vital structures. Therefore, tumor dissection should always be performed in a meticulous fashion. Because tumor bleeding can be extensive, complete visualization of the tumor extent is critical before extirpation is attempted. Cotton soaked with a hemostatic agent, bipolar electrocautery, and laser dissection can be useful tools for managing bleeding, although some debate exists regarding the best laser substrate.[47–50] The anterior portion of the tumor, adjacent to the petrous carotid artery, should generally be addressed last. Although preoperative CT helps to characterize the integrity of the carotid canal, palpation anteriorly should only be performed with a blunt-tipped instrument. Once the relationship of the tumor to the carotid artery has been established, dissection can proceed carefully. When freed from all vascular and ossicular attachments and the facial nerve, the tumor can usually be avulsed from the promontory, and hemostasis can be achieved using a laser, bipolar cautery, and/or gentle pressure with a cotton ball (Video 2). Once bleeding is controlled, the status of the ossicles and tympanic membrane is assessed, and tympanoplasty with ossiculoplasty should be performed if necessary.

Subtotal resection can be a consideration given the locally invasive tendencies of tympanic paragangliomas. Tumors can become attached to the ossicles, oval and round windows, dura, facial nerve, and petrous carotid artery. With regard to tumors attached to the petrous carotid artery, the authors identified 19.1% of patients with disease involving the eustachian tube and carotid artery. One patient (0.9%) with a recurrent class 4 tumor experienced a stroke during an attempt to resect adherent disease from this location. Subsequently, 7 patients had near-total resection with disease left on a vital structure, and no clinically significant progression has been seen in these patients after 44 months of follow-up.[34] Currently, the authors' preference is to leave limited adherent tumor remnants in place when complete excision risks morbidity to the facial nerve, carotid artery, or cochlea. These patients are then followed clinically and radiographically for surveillance of residual progressive disease.

Not all patients can tolerate general anesthesia, and nonsurgical management options can be considered if resection cannot be attempted. Given the slow-growing, benign nature of these tumors, observation with close clinical and radiologic follow-up can be used.[51] In the authors' experience, 7% of tumors were observed for an average of 25.5 months (median, 18 months), generally because of patient preference or unsuitability for general anesthesia.[34] Periodic reimaging and clinical evaluation can be sought on a yearly basis, with the possibility of extending the interval between scans if disease stability is demonstrated. Regarding the risks and benefits of watchful observation, the authors' experience highlights the generally indolent nature of tumor growth, because facial nerve injury and sensorineural hearing loss rarely occur in this setting.[34] When selecting a nonoperative approach, however, patients must be counseled that resection remains the gold standard for definitive management, and tumor growth can occasionally lead to irreversible facial weakness and/or sensorineural hearing loss, and episodic bloody otorrhea in cases of Glasscock-Jackson class 4 disease. Stereotactic radiation has also been described as a palliative measure for GT tumors,[52,53] although the authors only use this approach for growing tumors when no other options are available.

PROGNOSIS

With meticulous dissection and hemostasis, successful surgical resection of GT tumors can be performed with minimal morbidity. With regard to hearing outcomes, previous reports identify a trend toward improvement in air bone gap when tumor can be removed from the ossicular chain.[32,40] However, postoperative sensorineural loss can occur in some cases, particularly when tumor invasion of the cochleovestibular system has occurred via the oval or round windows or from a labyrinthine fistula.[32,34,40] Postoperative facial weakness is not commonly seen, although the likelihood is slightly higher with adherent disease when the facial nerve is extensively skeletonized or dehiscent during resection.[34] In addition to hearing loss and facial weakness, tympanic membrane perforation (1.7%), formation of acquired cholesteatoma (1.7%), surgical-site infection (1.7%), and cerebrospinal fluid leak (0.9%) are also possible but rare. Using the aforementioned approach, the authors saw no cases of disease recurrence through a mean follow-up of 30.4 months.[34]

SUMMARY

GT are paragangliomas of the middle ear cleft most commonly seen in middle-aged women. They are distinguished from glomus jugulare by the absence of bony erosion at the jugular foramen. Most tumors are benign and nonsecretory, but emerging data regarding the genetic basis of tumor formation suggest that certain patients are at higher risk for more aggressive, functional, and/or multicentric disease. Gross total resection is the only definitive therapy for these tumors, although subtotal excision is recommended when disease is adherent to vital structures in order to prevent unnecessary morbidity.

ACKNOWLEDGMENTS

The authors would like to thank Dr Katherine N. Kimmelshue (Department of Pathology, Vanderbilt University) for the images used in **Figs. 1** and **2**.

SUPPLEMENTARY DATA

Supplementary data related to this article can be found online at http://dx.doi.org/10.1016/j.otc.2014.12.004.

REFERENCES

1. Jackson CG, Leonetti JP, Marz SJ. Surgery for benign tumors of the temporal bone. Glasscock-Shambaugh surgery of the ear. In: Gulya AJ, Minor LB, Poe DS, editors. 6th edition. Shelton (CT): People's Medical Publishing House; 2010. p. 729–50.
2. Lingen MW, Kumar V. Head and neck. In: Kumar V, Abbas AK, Fausto N, editors. Robbins and Cotran pathologic basis of disease. 7th edition. Philadelphia: Elsevier Saunders; p. 773–96.
3. Boedeker CC, Ridder GJ, Schipper J. Paragangliomas of the head and neck: diagnosis and treatment. Fam Cancer 2005;4(1):55–9.
4. Weissman JL, Hirsch BE. Beyond the promontory: the multifocal origin of glomus tympanicum tumors. AJNR Am J Neuroradiol 1998;19:119–22.
5. Guild SR. A hitherto unrecognized structure, the glomus jugularis in man. Anat Rec 1941;79(Suppl 2):28.
6. Rosenwasser H. Carotid body tumor of the middle ear and mastoid. Arch Otolaryngol 1945;31:64.
7. Simpson IC, Dallachy R. A review of tumors of the glomus jugulare with reports to three further cases. J Laryngol Otol 1958;72:194–226.
8. Guild SR. Glomus jugularis in man. Ann Otol Rhinol Laryngol 1953;62:1045–71.
9. Alford BR, Guilford FR. A comprehensive study of tumors of the glomus jugulare. Laryngoscope 1962;72:765–805.
10. House WF, Glasscock ME III. Glomus tympanicum tumors. Arch Otolaryngol 1968;87:550–4.
11. Sennaroglu L, Sungur A. Histopathology of paragangliomas. Otol Neurotol 2002;23:104–5.
12. Kouzaki H, Fukui J, Shimizu T. Management of a catecholamine-secreting tympanicum glomus tumour: case report. J Laryngol Otol 2008;122:1377–80.
13. Schwaber MK, Glasscock ME, Jackson CG, et al. Diagnosis and management of catecholamine secreting glomus tumors. Laryngoscope 1984;94:1008–15.
14. Lawson W. The neuroendocrine nature of the glomus cells: an experimental, ultrastructural, and histochemical tissue culture study. Laryngoscope 1980;90:120–44.
15. Hirano S, Shoji K, Kojima H, et al. Dopamine-secreting carotid body tumor. Am J Otolaryngol 1998;19(6):412–6.
16. Parkinson D. Intracranial pheochromocytomas (active glomus jugulare). J Neurosurg 1969;31:94–100.
17. Duke WW, Boshen BR, Sotenes P. A norepinephrine-secreting glomus jugulare tumor presenting as a pheochromocytoma. Ann Intern Med 1964;60:1040–7.

18. Lee JH, Barich F, Karnell LH, et al. National cancer database report on malignant paragangliomas of the head and neck. Cancer 2002;94:730-7.

19. Manolidis S, Shohet JA, Jackson CG, et al. Malignant glomus tumors. Laryngoscope 1999;109:30-4.

20. Borsanyi SJ. Glomus jugulare tumors. Laryngoscope 1962;72:1336-45.

21. Kahn LB. Vagal body tumor (nonchromaffin paraganglioma, chemodectoma and carotid body-like tumor) with cervical node metastasis and familial association. Ultrastructural study and review. Cancer 1976;38:2367-77.

22. Lattes R, Waltner JG. Nonchromaffin paraganglioma of the middle ear. Cancer 1948;2:447-68.

23. Martin TP, Irving RM, Maher ER. The genetics of paragangliomas: a review. Clin Otolaryngol 2007;32(1):7-11.

24. Mariman EC, van Beersum SE, Cremers CW, et al. Fine mapping of a putatively imprinted gene for familial non-chromaffin paragangliomas to chromosome 11q13.1: evidence for genetic heterogeneity. Hum Genet 1995;95:56-62.

25. Bikhazi PH, Messina L, Mhatre AN, et al. Molecular pathogenesis in sporadic head and neck paraganglioma. Laryngoscope 2000;110:1346-8.

26. Devilee P, van Schothorst EM, Bardoel AF, et al. Allelotype of head and neck paragangliomas: allelic imbalance is confined to the long arm of chromosome 11, the site of the predisposing locus PGL. Genes Chromosomes Cancer 1994; 11(2):71-8.

27. Pellitteri P, Rinaldo A, Myssiorek D, et al. Paragangliomas of the head and neck. Oral Oncol 2004;40:563-75.

28. Niemann S, Muller U. Mutations in SDHC cause autosomal dominant paraganglioma. Nat Genet 2000;26:268-70.

29. Neumann HP, Pawlu C, Peczkowska M, et al. Distinct clinical features of paraganglioma syndromes associated with SDHB and SDHD gene mutations. JAMA 2004;292:943-51.

30. Schiavi F, Boedeker CC, Bausch B, et al. Predictors and prevalence of paraganglioma syndrome associated with mutations of the SDHC gene. JAMA 2005; 294(16):2057-63.

31. Boedeker CC, Neumann HP, Maier W, et al. Malignant head and neck paragangliomas in SDHB mutation carriers. Otolaryngol Head Neck Surg 2007;137:126-9.

32. O'Leary MJ, Shelton C, Giddings NA, et al. Glomus tympanicum tumors: a clinical perspective. Laryngoscope 1991;101:1038-43.

33. Sanna M, Fois P, Pasanisi E, et al. Middle ear and mastoid glomus tumors (glomus tympanicum): an algorithm for the surgical management. Auris Nasus Larynx 2010;37(6):661-8.

34. Carlson ML, Sweeney AD, Pelosi S, et al. Surgical management of glomus tympanicum: a review of 115 cases over four decades. Otolaryngol Head Neck Surg 2015;152:136-42.

35. Jacobs IN, Potsic WP. Glomus tympanicum in infancy. Arch Otolaryngol Head Neck Surg 1994;120:203-5.

36. Hirunpat S, Riabroi K, Dechsukhum C, et al. Nasopharyngeal extension of glomus tympanicum: an unusual clinical and imaging manifestation. AJNR Am J Neuroradiol 2006;27:1820-2.

37. McKiever ME, Carlson ML, Neff BA. Aberrant petrous carotid artery masquerading as a glomus tympanicum. Otol Neurotol 2014;35:e228-30.

38. Wanna GB, Sweeney AD, Carlson ML, et al. Subtotal resection for management of large jugular paragangliomas with functional lower cranial nerves. Otolaryngol Head Neck Surg 2014;151(6):991-5.

39. Carlson ML, Sweeney AD, Wanna GB, et al. Natural history of glomus jugulare: a review of 16 tumors managed with primary observation. Otolaryngol Head Neck Surg 2015;152:98–105.
40. Jackson CG, Welling DB, Chironis P, et al. Glomus tympanicum tumors: contemporary concepts in conservation surgery. Laryngoscope 1999;99:875–84.
41. Fisch U. Infratemporal fossa approach for extensive tumors of the temporal bone and base of skull. In: Silverstein H, Norrell H, editors. Neurological surgery of the ear. Birmingham (AL): Aesculapius; 1977. p. 34–53.
42. van Houtum WH, Corssmit EP, Douwes Decker PB, et al. Increased prevalaence of catecholamine excess and phaeochromocytomas in a well-defined Dutch population with SDHD-linked head and neck paragangliomas. Eur J Endocrinol 2005;152(1):87–94.
43. Sridhara SK, Yener M, Hanna EY, et al. Genetic testing in head and neck paraganglioma: who, what, and why? J Neurol Surg B Skull Base 2013;74(4): 236–40.
44. Neumann HP, Erlic Z, Boedeker CC, et al. Clinical predictors for germline mutations in head and neck paraganglioma patients: cost reduction strategy in genetic diagnostic process as fall-out. Cancer Res 2009;69(8):3650–6.
45. Colen TY, Mihm FG, Mason TP, et al. Catecholamine-secreting paragangliomas: recent progress in diagnosis and perioperative management. Skull Base 2009; 19(6):377–85.
46. Papaspyrou K, Mewes T, Tóth M, et al. Hearing results after hypotympanotomy for glomus tympanicum tumors. Otol Neurotol 2011;32(2):291–6.
47. Durvasula VS, De R, Baguley DM, et al. Laser excision of glomus tympanicum tumours: long-term results. Eur Arch Otorhinolaryngol 2005;262(4):325–7.
48. Molony NC, Salto-Tellez M, Grant WE. KTP laser assisted excision of glomus tympanicum. J Laryngol Otol 1998;112(10):956–8.
49. Robinson PJ, Grant HR, Bown SG. NdYAG laser treatment of a glomus tympanicum tumour. J Laryngol Otol 1993;107(3):236–7.
50. Jovanovic S. Lasers in otology. In: Hüttenbrink KB, editor. Lasers in otorhinolaryngology. New York: Thieme; 2005. p. 21–52.
51. Cosetti M, Linstrom C, Alexiades G, et al. Glomus tumors in patients of advanced age: a conservative approach. Laryngoscope 2008;118(2):270–4.
52. Lee C, Pan DH, Wu JC, et al. Gamma knife radiosurgery for glomus jugulare and tympanicum. Stereotact Funct Neurosurg 2011;89(5):291–8.
53. Gilbo P, Morris CG, Amdur RJ, et al. Radiotherapy for benign head and neck paragangliomas: a 45-year experience. Cancer 2014. http://dx.doi.org/10.1002/cncr.28923s.

Adenomatous Tumors of the Middle Ear

Stanley Pelosi, MD[a],*, Shira Koss, MD[b]

KEYWORDS

- Adenomatous middle ear tumor • Middle ear adenoma • Middle ear carcinoid
- Mixed adenoma • Neuroendocrine adenoma • Amphicrine tumor

KEY POINTS

- Adenomatous middle ear tumors can present with a variety of symptoms, most commonly conductive hearing loss.
- Clinical diagnosis of adenomatous middle ear tumors is complex because they may show significant overlap with other entities, such as paraganglioma.
- There is no imaging study to definitively diagnose adenomatous middle ear tumors, but computed tomography and MRI can be useful.
- Classification of adenomatous middle ear tumors is controversial and there is much debate over whether middle ear adenoma and carcinoid represent two ends of the same spectrum or distinct entities.
- Management of adenomatous middle ear tumors is surgical, involving a tympanoplasty or tympanomastoidectomy; in monitoring for recurrence, clinical examination alone may be appropriate for patients with limited disease at the time of initial surgery, whereas more aggressive tumors may also necessitate imaging.

OVERVIEW

Adenomatous tumors are an uncommon cause of a middle ear mass. The first description of middle ear adenoma as a distinct pathologic entity was by Hyams and Michaels[1] in 1976, who described a series of 20 glandular middle ear neoplasms that did not resemble paraganglioma or salivary gland tumor.[1] In the same year, Derlacki and Barney[2] reported on 3 additional cases with similar histopathology.[2] Murphy and colleagues[3] in 1980 then described a middle ear tumor with related pathologic features but additionally having histochemical and ultrastructural evidence of neuroendocrine differentiation, labeling it carcinoid. Other investigators have subsequently reported similarly behaving middle ear tumors using the term neuroendocrine

Disclosures: The authors have no disclosures or conflicts of interest.
^a Department of Otolaryngology - Head and Neck Surgery, Thomas Jefferson University, 925 Chestnut Street, 6th Floor, Philadelphia, PA 19107, USA; ^b Department of Otolaryngology - Head and Neck Surgery, The New York Eye and Ear Infirmary, 310 East 14th Street, New York, NY 10024, USA
* Corresponding author.
E-mail address: stanley.pelosi@jefferson.edu

Otolaryngol Clin N Am 48 (2015) 305–315
http://dx.doi.org/10.1016/j.otc.2014.12.005
0030-6665/15/$ – see front matter © 2015 Elsevier Inc. All rights reserved.

adenoma.[4,5] Recent histopathologic evidence suggests that such labels may represent a spectrum of 1 common pathologic entity.[6] In contrast, other researchers still posit that middle ear adenoma and carcinoid are distinct biological neoplasms.[7,8]

The commonality to all adenomatous middle ear tumors is the presence of both epithelial and neuroendocrine elements. Immunohistochemical staining shows 2 distinct patterns of staining; one for cytokeratin markers within the glandular components of the tumor and another for neuroendocrine markers in the stromal regions.[6] Similarly, electron microscopy can be used to reveal ultrastructural features within adenomatous tumors that confirm the presence of these opposing cell types.

Most adenomatous middle ear tumors show indolent biological behavior, with a benign histologic appearance and slow local growth. More aggressive histologic patterns may also sometimes be observed, although uncertainty exists as to whether this predicts an increased risk of local invasiveness, recurrence, and/or metastasis. Examples have been cited of locally invasive tumors that appear histologically benign as well as neoplasms that contain infiltrative/dysplastic cellular morphologies but do not show clinical invasiveness.[2,9] Because of the rarity of adenomatous middle ear tumors, along with uncertainties in classification and differences in biological behavior, rigid protocols for management of these tumors are lacking.

CLINICAL PRESENTATION

Adenomatous middle ear tumor typically presents as a nonspecific middle ear mass (**Fig. 1**). The mean age of presentation is the fifth decade (range, 14–80 years)[10] with no gender preference.[11] Hearing loss was the most common presenting symptom (86.3%) in a review of 94 previously published cases of middle ear glandular neoplasms, with most being conductive in nature. Other reported symptoms included aural fullness (33%), tinnitus (27.6%), otalgia (15%), otorrhea (11.4%), and facial weakness (11%).[11] Facial nerve palsies associated with middle ear tumors have been reported by Krouse and colleagues[12] and Torske and Thompson.[6] There was no nerve infiltration by tumor in any of these cases. Instead, the palsies were thought to be related to anatomic abnormalities or local pressure from the tumor with facial canal bone dehiscence.[6,12] Gross facial nerve invasion has been described in 1 case of

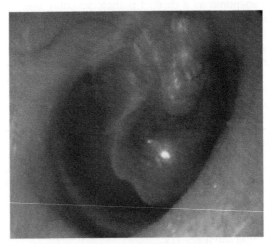

Fig. 1. Otomicroscopy of a right ear shows a middle ear mass medial to an intact tympanic membrane. (*Courtesy of* Matthew Carlson, MD, Rochester, MN.)

middle ear carcinoid and presumed in another case, as reported by Ramsey and colleagues.[8]

Regional and/or systemic symptoms may occasionally be associated with adenomatous middle ear tumors. There has been a case reported of middle ear carcinoid metastatic to ipsilateral cervical lymph nodes.[13] Also of note, a carcinoid tumor of the middle ear associated with carcinoid syndrome was described in 1980 by Farrior and colleagues[14] and in 1987 by Latif and colleagues.[15] In the latter report, the patient presented with systemic signs and symptoms including diarrhea, abdominal cramps, skin flushing, and bronchoconstriction.[15]

DIAGNOSIS

The differential diagnosis of middle ear masses is extensive and includes chronic otitis media, cholesteatoma, mucosal adenoma, ceruminous adenoma, carcinoid, paraganglioma, adenoid cystic carcinoma, pleomorphic adenoma, meningioma, schwannoma, retrotympanic vascular masses, endolymphatic sac tumor, schneiderian-type mucosal papilloma, lipoma, and epidermoid.[5,7,16] Adenomatous middle ear tumors can be distinguished based on several imaging and histologic characteristics.

IMAGING

Preoperative evaluation includes use of computed tomography (CT) and MRI to delineate tumor features. CT highlights a nonspecific opacity with possible extension to the tympanic cavity and mastoid (**Fig. 2**). The ossicles are generally embedded in the mass without ossicular or bony erosion or destruction. No characteristic differences between benign and malignant adenomatous middle ear tumors are detectable on CT.

MRI may be helpful in cases with extension to the posterior or middle cranial fossa.[16,17] On MRI, tumors are isointense to hyperintense relative to white matter on T1-weighted images, and avidly enhance with gadolinium administration (**Fig. 3**). On T2-weighted images, tumors approximate the signal intensity of gray matter.

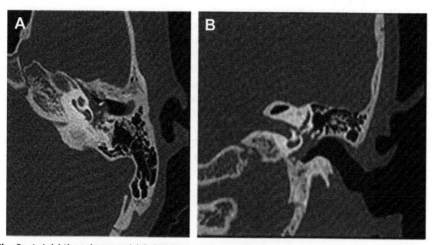

Fig. 2. Axial (A) and coronal (B) CT images of a middle ear adenoma, showing a nonspecific middle ear mass with ossicular chain involvement. (*Courtesy of* Dr David S. Haynes, Nashville, TN.)

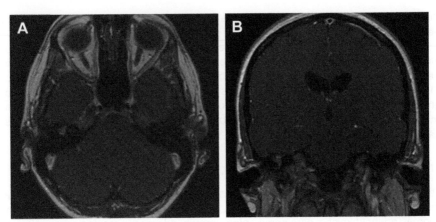

Fig. 3. Axial (*A*) and coronal (*B*) T1-weighted magnetic resonance images of a middle ear adenoma, showing an enhancing middle ear mass. (*Courtesy of* Matthew Carlson, MD, Rochester, MN.)

As previously noted, paraganglioma is an important consideration in the differential diagnosis of adenomatous middle ear tumors. Bierry and colleagues[18] presented several radiologic and clinical findings to help discriminate between these disorders; the investigators included carcinoid and noncarcinoid tumors under the term middle ear adenoma. They concluded that although middle ear adenomas and glomus tympanicum both appear as tissular lesions with significant enhancement on CT and MRI, only glomus tumors have specific clinical features such as pulsatile tinnitus, a close relationship between tumor and Jacobson nerve or its branches, and vascular blush on angiography. In contrast, adenomatous middle ear tumors are clearly separate from the Jacobson nerve and its branches, and although they show contrast enhancement, they have unimpressive angiographic findings. The study discussed use of conventional angiography in differentiating tumor types, but not CT or magnetic resonance angiography.

Evaluation of patients with suspected metastases (neck mass, systemic symptoms) should include imaging of the neck, chest, and abdomen. Octreotide scanning has been successfully used for localizing undetected primary or metastatic gastroenteropancreatic carcinoid disease with a sensitivity of 80% to 90%,[19] but is not well established in middle ear carcinoid and is limited to a single 2004 case report by Nikanne and colleagues.[20] Postoperative octreotide scan was used in this case because of a positive tumor margin near the eustachian tube; slight immediate postoperative uptake was thought to be caused by inflammation and repeat scan 4 months later was within normal limits. The investigators concluded that octreotide scanning is a sensitive method for follow-up in cases of both middle ear carcinoid recurrence and metastases.[20] No studies have assessed the use of diagnostic and preoperative octreotide scanning for these tumors.

PATHOGENESIS

The precursor cell for adenomatous middle ear tumors is unclear. Hyams and Michaels[1] postulated an origin for middle ear adenoma from surface epithelium mucosa, as did Derlacki and Barney.[2] It has also been suggested that middle ear adenomas develop from displaced or trapped embryonic rests of glandular cells in middle ear mucosa,[7] and some investigators have suggested that these embryonic cells are of neural crest origin.[6]

Other reports have deemphasized the relationship between middle ear adenoma and neuroendocrine tumors, maintaining that they are separate entities.[21] The middle ear does not contain enterochromaffin cells, which normally give rise to carcinoid tumors in the lung and gastrointestinal tract, nor does it contain other cells with neuroendocrine features. One potential explanation put forth by Torske and Thompson[6] is that an undifferentiated, pluripotent stem cell may give rise to an adenomatous middle ear tumor with both epithelial and neuroendocrine components.

Carcinoids are rare in the middle ear and mastoid. The tumor occurs predominantly in the small intestine, and, when these lesions develop in the head and neck region, most arise in the larynx.[22,23] The first case of middle ear carcinoid was reported in 1980 by Murphy and colleagues[3] and in 2005 Chan and colleagues[24] found approximately 40 cases of documented middle ear carcinoid in the English literature. Carcinoid has historically been considered a distinct neoplasm given its reported metastatic potential.[8,13,25] However, recent studies have used pathologic features to suggest that middle ear adenoma and carcinoid may represent different stages of differentiation of the same tumor. Hence many investigators currently view these tumors as a single primary low-grade glandular neoplasm, with more specific identification based on immunohistochemical markers and presence or absence of metastases.[6,11,26]

MICROSCOPY AND IMMUNOHISTOCHEMISTRY

On light microscopy, middle ear adenomas and carcinoid tumors have been described with similar, often indistinguishable, morphologies.[27–29] Although predominant architectural patterns can vary both between and within the same tumor, they are often arranged in glandular spaces, trabeculae, festoons, ribbonlike patterns, anastomosing cords, and solid sheets (**Fig. 4**). In both neoplasms, the cells are described as cuboidal to columnar; uniform in size; with eosinophilic, finely granular cytoplasm. The nuclei are round to oval with finely dispersed chromatin and may be centrally or eccentrically located with a plasmacytoid appearance sometimes noted on electron microscopy.[30] Nucleoli are inconspicuous and mitoses are almost never present. They may be distinguished from paraganglioma in that the paraganglioma contain richly vascularized stroma and characteristic zellballen pattern.

Classically, endocrine synthetic activity is reflected by the presence of cytoplasmic neurosecretory granules on light microscopy and specific positive immunohistochemical staining of neuroendocrine cells.[25] However, immunohistochemical staining for both middle ear adenomas and neuroendocrine carcinoid tumors has shown similar results.[29–32] In both, the glandular spaces commonly contain secretory product that stains with mucicarmine, periodic acid–Schiff, and Alcian blue.[30] Both tumors are also positive for a variety of markers including cytokeratin cocktail and vimentin immunostaining; neuroendocrine markers such as neuron-specific enolase, chromogranin, and synaptophysin have also been uniformly present in both tumors, although not necessarily all in the same tumor. In one study, human pancreatic polypeptide was almost uniformly positive, and in both tumors variable positivity for S-100, serotonin, glucagon, Leu-7, adrenocorticotropic hormone, and somatostatin has been noted.[6]

In multiple studies, the location and degree of positivity of the immunohistochemical staining varied with architectural pattern. Cytokeratin was most strongly identified in the cytoplasm of the glandular component and weakest in the solid component.[32,33] Neuroendocrine markers were most strongly identified in the trabecular, ribbon, and

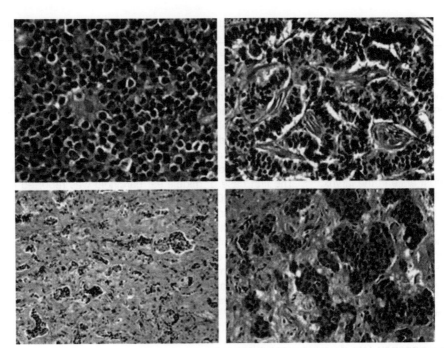

Fig. 4. Pathologic examination of adenomatous middle ear tumors using hematoxylin and eosin stains may show multiple architectural patterns. (*From* Torske KR, Thompson LD. Adenoma versus carcinoid tumor of the middle ear: a study of 48 cases and review of the literature. Mod Pathol 2002;15:543–55, with permission.)

solid components, and only weakly shown in the glandular component, except for keratin 7, which was glandular specific.[32,34]

Immunohistochemical staining can be a useful tool in differentiating adenomatous middle ear tumors from other neuroendocrine tumors, such as paraganglioma. The absence of S-100 protein positivity, combined with strong positive staining for keratin, strongly argues against a diagnosis of paraganglioma. Immunostaining for galanin may also be useful because carcinoid tumors have proved to be galanin negative, whereas some paragangliomas have been found to be galanin positive.[25,35]

Aggressive histologic subtypes of middle ear adenoma have been reported, but their existence has been called into question based on the histologic and gross behavioral resemblance to endolymphatic sac tumors. Endolymphatic sac tumors contain neoplastic cells with adenomatous features arranged in papillary configurations, and were first recognized as a distinct biological entity in 1989.[36] Several clinical series predating this report have described aggressive middle ear papillary adenoma[37] or adenocarcinoma[38,39] causing significant bony destruction and facial nerve or posterior fossa involvement, behavior that is also characteristic of endolymphatic sac tumors. The shared pathologic features and aggressive clinical presentation suggests that these aggressive tumors are more likely to be endolymphatic sac tumors than variants of middle ear adenoma.

CLASSIFICATION

No generally accepted classification system exists in the literature for adenomatous middle ear tumors. One recently proposed scheme was described by Saliba and

Evrard,[11] who classified middle ear glandular neoplasms into 3 subtypes. The most common neoplasm (type I) is the neuroendocrine adenoma of the middle ear, which shows positive immunohistochemistry and negative metastasis. A type II tumor is the middle ear adenoma, which shows negative immunohistochemistry and negative metastasis. The least common type (type III) within this classification scheme is the carcinoid tumor of the middle ear, which shows positive immunohistochemistry and positive metastasis and/or carcinoid syndrome.

TREATMENT

The management of adenomatous middle ear tumors is surgical, with operative approach dictated by the extent of disease. A transcanal approach can be used for small tumors limited to the mesotympanum, or for tumors extending through the tympanic membrane into the external auditory canal. Access for larger tumors with extension to the epitympanum and/or mastoid can be accomplished with a tympanoplasty and intact canal wall mastoidectomy. One review of 94 previously reported adenomatous middle ear tumors found that 15% of tumors extended to the mastoid.[11] Achieving access for removal may require an extended facial recess or canal wall down approach. Perforation of the tympanic membrane with extension into the external auditory canal is a feature that is occasionally identified,[28] and may require canalplasty along with tympanic membrane repair. A translabyrinthine route is rarely used for tumors that erode the otic capsule and result in profound hearing loss. Macroscopically, adenomatous middle ear tumors have been described as soft, rubbery masses that are not encapsulated. Lesions may be several colors, including gray-tan,[2] brown-red,[1] or pale yellow.[6]

Whenever possible, complete excision is preferred. The ossicular chain is frequently involved with disease (**Fig. 5**); Ramsey and colleagues[8] reported 72% of middle ear carcinoids to have ossicular involvement. In such cases the ossicles are generally removed and reconstruction performed, although one report also described that repeated debulking procedures preserved the ossicular chain.[6] True ossicle destruction was rare in other studies.[28,40]

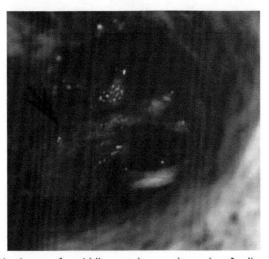

Fig. 5. Intraoperative image of a middle ear adenoma (*arrowhead*) adjacent to the malleus. (*Courtesy of* Dr David S. Haynes, Nashville, TN.)

As described previously, facial paresis may be a symptom associated with carcinoid tumors. Most cases involving facial weakness do not report nerve infiltration by tumor, although gross facial nerve invasion has occasionally been described.[8] Subtotal resection may be a consideration in cases in which tumor is intimately associated with the facial nerve so as to avoid iatrogenic injury. Regional metastatic disease may be managed surgically with a parotidectomy and/or neck dissection.

Adjuvant treatment of adenomatous middle ear tumors with radiation or chemotherapy is generally not recommended. Radiation has occasionally been described for treatment of middle ear carcinoids but is not thought to improve control rates.[8] One report described metastatic spread following adjuvant radiation in a patient with middle ear carcinoid.[13]

OUTCOME/PROGNOSIS

Torske and Thompson[6] summarized outcomes of a series of 48 patients with adenomatous middle ear tumors. With a mean follow-up of more than 15 years, the overall recurrence rate was 18%. Similarly, Ramsey and colleagues[8] reported a recurrence rate of 22% for carcinoid tumors. Several factors have been proposed to affect recurrence, one being surgical approach. Ramsey and colleagues[8] found the rate of recurrence in carcinoid tumors to be higher in patients undergoing transcanal removal versus canal wall down mastoidectomy, although this difference did not reach statistical significance.[8]

In addition, management of the ossicles may play a role in recurrent disease, with an increased likelihood in cases with ossicular involvement in which the ossicular chain is not removed.[6] A review by Saliba and Evrard[11] corroborated these findings, reporting that in all patients with recurrence the ossicular chain had been left intact at initial surgery.

It is unclear whether intrinsic tumor biology affects recurrence rates. Of the 8 patients with recurrence in the Torske and Thompson[6] series, 2 had moderate cellular pleomorphism on histologic examination, and another 2 had high cellularity. Likewise,

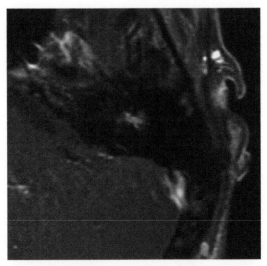

Fig. 6. Axial MRI showing an enhancing mass in the middle ear cavity suspicious for recurrent middle ear adenoma. (*Courtesy of* Dr David S. Haynes, Nashville, TN.)

metastatic disease is not necessarily associated with high-grade disorder. Ramsey and colleagues[8] found that all cases of carcinoid recurrence were associated with well-differentiated neoplasms.

A few cases of primary carcinoid tumors of the middle ear with metastases have been reported. In 1999, Mooney and colleagues[13] reported a 64-year old man with a 9-year history of a recurring middle ear neoplasm and ipsilateral cervical lymphadenopathy. In addition, in 2005, Ramsey and colleagues[8] described 2 cases of primary middle ear carcinoid with late recurrences and regional metastases. To date, distant metastases from middle ear carcinoid have not been reported.[25] The lack of documented distant metastasis of middle ear tumors may be explained by both the small size of the neoplasms and the lack of vascularity of the middle ear cavity.

Long-term follow-up is recommended for all patients, although no consensus exists regarding an optimal surveillance schedule. Clinical examination alone may be appropriate for benign lesions with limited disease at the time of initial surgery, although for more aggressive tumors otomicroscopy combined with CT and/or MRI can be used to monitor for recurrence (**Fig. 6**).

SUMMARY

Adenomatous tumors of the middle ear should be recognized by the otologic surgeon as a rare cause of middle ear mass. They most commonly present with conductive hearing loss, and appear on imaging as nonspecific soft tissue masses involving the middle ear and/or mastoid. Surgery is the recommended treatment strategy, with surgical approach dictated by extent of disease. Accurate recognition of adenomatous middle ear tumors allows prompt management and limitation of morbidity.

REFERENCES

1. Hyams VJ, Michaels L. Benign adenomatous neoplasm (adenoma) of the middle ear. Clin Otolaryngol Allied Sci 1976;1:17–26.
2. Derlacki EL, Barney PL. Adenomatous tumors of the middle ear and mastoid. Laryngoscope 1976;86:1123–35.
3. Murphy GF, Pilch BZ, Dickersin GR, et al. Carcinoid tumor of the middle ear. Am J Clin Pathol 1980;73:816–23.
4. Aquino BF, Chandra RK, Haines GK, et al. Neuroendocrine adenoma of the middle ear. Otolaryngol Head Neck Surg 2002;127(5):477–9.
5. Leong K, Haber MM, Divi V, et al. Neuroendocrine adenoma of the middle ear (NAME). Ear Nose Throat J 2009;88:874–9.
6. Torske KR, Thompson LD. Adenoma versus carcinoid tumor of the middle ear: a study of 48 cases and review of the literature. Mod Pathol 2002;15:543–55.
7. Wackym PA, Friedman I. Unusual tumors of the middle ear and mastoid. In: Jackler RJ, Driscoll CL, editors. Tumors of the middle ear and temporal bone. Philadelphia: Lippincott Williams and Wilkins; 2000. p. 128–45.
8. Ramsey MJ, Nadol JB, Pilch BZ, et al. Carcinoid tumor of the middle ear: clinical features, recurrences, and metastases. Laryngoscope 2005;115:1660–6.
9. Pallanch JF, Weiland LH, McDonald TJ, et al. Adenocarcinoma and adenoma of the middle ear. Laryngoscope 1982;92:47–54.
10. Ayache S, Braccini F, Fernandes M, et al. Adenoma of the middle ear: a rare and misleading lesion. Otol Neurotol 2002;23(6):988–91.
11. Saliba I, Evrard AS. Middle ear glandular neoplasms: adenoma, carcinoma or adenoma with neuroendocrine differentiation: a case series. Cases J 2009;2:6508.

12. Krouse JH, Nadol JB Jr, Goodman ML. Carcinoid tumors of the middle ear. Ann Otol Rhinol Laryngol 1990;99:547–52.
13. Mooney EE, Dodd LG, Oury TD, et al. Middle ear carcinoid: an indolent tumor with metastatic potential. Head Neck 1999;21:72–7.
14. Farrior JB 3rd, Hyams VJ, Benke RH, et al. Carcinoid apudoma arising in a glomus jugulare tumor: review of endocrine activity in glomus jugulare tumors. Laryngoscope 1980;90:110–9.
15. Latif MA, Madders DJ, Barton RP, et al. Carcinoid tumour of the middle ear associated with systemic symptoms. J Laryngol Otol 1987;101:4.
16. Zan E, Limb CJ, Koehler JF, et al. Middle ear adenoma: a challenging diagnosis. AJNR Am J Neuroradiol 2009;30:1602–3.
17. Maintz D, Stupp C, Krueger K, et al. MRI and CT of adenomatous tumours of the middle ear. Neuroradiology 2001;43(1):58–61.
18. Bierry G, Riehm S, Marcellin L, et al. Middle ear adenomatous tumor: a not so rare glomus tympanicum-mimicking lesion. J Neuroradiol 2010;37:116–21.
19. Krenning EP, Kwekkeboom DJ, Oei HY, et al. Somatostatin-receptor scintigraphy in gastroenteropancreatic tumors. An overview of European results. Ann N Y Acad Sci 1994;733:416–24.
20. Nikanne E, Kantola O, Parvianinen T. Carcinoid tumor of middle ear. Duodecim 2003;119:1081–4.
21. Friedmann I. Middle ear adenoma. Histopathology 1998;32(3):279–80.
22. Soga J, Ferlito A, Rinaldo A. Endocrinocarcinomas (carcinoids and their variants) of the larynx: a comparative consideration with those of other sites. Oral Oncol 2004;40:668–72.
23. Ferlito A, Rinaldo A. The spectrum of endocrinocarcinomas of the larynx. Oral Oncol 2005;41:878–83.
24. Chan KC, Wu CM, Huang SF. Carcinoid tumor of the middle ear: a case report. Am J Otolaryngol 2005;26:57–9.
25. Ferlito A, Devaney KO, Rinaldo A. Neuroendocrine neoplasms of the larynx: advances in identification, understanding, and management. Oral Oncol 2006; 42(8):770–88.
26. Cruz Toro P, Domenech I, Clemente I, et al. Temporal bone histopathology case of the month neuroendocrine adenoma of the middle ear. Otol Neurotol 2011;33: e7–8.
27. Mills SE, Fechner RE. Middle ear adenoma. A cytologically uniform neoplasm displaying a variety of architectural patterns. Am J Surg Pathol 1984;8:677–85.
28. Hosoda S, Tateno H, Inoue HK, et al. Carcinoid tumor of the middle ear containing serotonin and multiple peptide hormones. A case report and review of the pathology literature. Acta Pathol Jpn 1992;42:614–20.
29. Manni JJ, Faverly DR, Van Haelst UJ. Primary carcinoid tumors of the middle ear. Report on four cases and a review of the literature. Arch Otolaryngol Head Neck Surg 1992;118:1341–7.
30. Ribe A, Fernandez PL, Ostertarg H, et al. Middle-ear adenoma (MEA): a report of two cases, one with predominant "plasmacytoid" features. Histopathology 1997; 30:359–64.
31. Ketabchi S, Massi D, Franchi A, et al. Middle ear adenoma is an amphicrine tumor: why call it adenoma? Ultrastruct Pathol 2001;25:73–8.
32. Paraskevakou H, Lazaris AC, Kandiloros DC, et al. Middle ear adenomatous tumor with a predominant neuroendocrine component. Pathology 1999;31:284–7.
33. Stanley MW, Horowitz CA, Levinson RM, et al. Carcinoid tumors of the middle ear. Am J Clin Pathol 1987;87:592–600.

34. Wassef M, Kanavaros P, Nemeth J, et al. Amphicrine adenoma of the middle ear. Histological, immunohistochemical and ultrastructural study of a case. Ann Pathol 1993;13(3):170–5.
35. Tadros TS, Strauss RM, Cohen C, et al. Galanin immunoreactivity in paragangliomas but not in carcinoid tumors. Appl Immunohistochem Mol Morphol 2003;11: 250–2.
36. Heffner DK. Low-grade adenocarcinoma of probable endolymphatic sac origin: a clinicopathologic study of 20 cases. Cancer 1989;64:2292–302.
37. Gaffey MJ, Mills SE, Fechner RE, et al. Progressive papillary middle ear tumor. A clinicopathologic entity distinct from middle-ear adenoma. Am J Surg Pathol 1988;12:790–7.
38. Fayemi AO, Toker C. Primary adenocarcinoma of the middle ear. Arch Otolaryngol 1975;101:449–52.
39. Schuller DE, Conley JJ, Goodman JH, et al. Primary adenocarcinoma of the middle ear. Otolaryngol Head Neck Surg 1983;91(3):280–3.
40. Hardingham M. Adenoma of the middle ear. Arch Otolaryngol Head Neck Surg 1995;121:342–4.

Endolymphatic Sac Tumors

Cameron C. Wick, MD[a], Nauman F. Manzoor, MD[a],
Maroun T. Semaan, MD[a,b], Cliff A. Megerian, MD[a,b],*

KEYWORDS

- Endolymphatic sac tumors • Von Hippel–Lindau • Hearing preservation
- Meniere syndrome

KEY POINTS

- Endolymphatic sac tumors (ELST) are slow-growing, locally aggressive, low-grade malignancies that originate from the epithelium of the endolymphatic duct and sac.
- Common presenting symptoms are asymmetrical sensorineural hearing loss, tinnitus, and vertigo, which may mimic Meniere disease.
- There is a well-established link between von Hippel–Lindau disease and ELST.
- Microsurgical excision, possibly via a retrolabyrinthine–transdural approach, is the treatment of choice.
- Early diagnosis may enable hearing preservation and cochlear implants may also restore hearing provided the cochlear nerve is intact.

BACKGROUND

Endolymphatic sac tumors (ELST) are slow-growing, locally aggressive, low-grade malignancies that originate from the epithelium of the endolymphatic duct and sac. Adenomatous tumors of the temporal bone have gone through a variety of classification schemes. In 1957, it was recognized that adenomas and adenocarcinomas of the external auditory canal originated in the apocrine glands of the canal, thus the term "ceruminoma" was coined.[1] The origin of primary adenomatous tumors within the middle ear cleft was debated, with some authors supporting aberrant ceruminous glands and others postulating that the tumors arise from native middle ear mucosa.[2,3]

Disclosures: The authors have no financial disclosures relevant to this topic.
[a] Ear, Nose, and Throat Institute, University Hospitals Case Medical Center, Case Western Reserve University School of Medicine, Cleveland, OH, USA; [b] Otology, Neurotology, and Balance Disorders, Department of Otolaryngology – Head and Neck Surgery, Ear, Nose, and Throat Institute, University Hospitals Case Medical Center, Case Western Reserve University School of Medicine, Cleveland, OH, USA
* Corresponding author.
E-mail address: Cliff.Megerian@UHhospitals.org

Otolaryngol Clin N Am 48 (2015) 317–330
http://dx.doi.org/10.1016/j.otc.2014.12.006
0030-6665/15/$ – see front matter © 2015 Elsevier Inc. All rights reserved.

oto.theclinics.com

In 1988, Gaffey and colleagues[4] recognized a particularly aggressive variant of "low-grade papillary adenocarcinoma" in the temporal bone that exhibited hypervascularity and local invasion with bony destruction. Shortly after, Heffner[5] reviewed 20 cases with similar papillary architecture and an epicenter at the posteromedial petrous bone where the endolymphatic sac resides. It was Heffner who suggested a link between this aggressive adenocarcinoma variant and the endolymphatic sac, which he termed "adenocarcinoma of the endolymphatic sac."[5] The notion of a tumor arising from the endolymphatic sac was supported by a report from Hassard and colleagues[6] in 1984 of a small, adenomatous sac lesion encountered during decompression surgery for suspected Meniere disease. In 1993, Li and colleagues[7] proposed a reclassification of these aggressive adenomatous lesions to ELST.

Still, the origin of ELST was debated. The clinical distinction between ELST from adenocarcinoma of the middle ear, metastasis, or choroid plexus tumors was often difficult.[8–12] In 1995, Megerian and colleagues[13] reviewed the Massachusetts Eye and Ear Infirmary's temporal bone collection and identified 8 specimens consistent with an aggressive papillary tumor of the temporal bone. All patients had sensorineural hearing loss (SNHL) and many had a Meniere-like presentation. One patient, a 48-year-old man with von Hippel–Lindau (VHL) disease, had succumbed to what was believed to be metastatic renal cell carcinoma to the left temporal bone. Upon further review, this tumor was more consistent with an ELST. Fortuitously, in this patient's contralateral temporal bone, a small de novo lesion within the endolymphatic sac was also identified and was histologically identical to the destructive lesion on the left (**Fig. 1**). This study validated that the epithelium of the endolymphatic sac was capable of producing a low-grade, locally aggressive papillary lesion. It also solidified a predilection for ELST in patients with VHL disease.[13] Subsequently, differences in immunohistochemistry staining patterns between ELST and choroid plexus tumors helped to distinguish these 2 disease entities. Specifically, choroid plexus tumors stain strongly with transthyretin (prealbumin), whereas ELST do not.[14] The confirmation of the origin of ELST and the recognition of sporadic versus VHL-related tumors enabled a better appreciation of the tumor's behavior, a staging system, and advancements in management as described herein.

CLINICAL PRESENTATION

ELST are rare tumors with approximately 200 cases reported in the literature. The true incidence of these tumors is unknown. Sporadic ELST are more common than those associated with VHL disease and have been diagnosed over a wide age range (15–77 years old) with the average diagnosis occurring in the fifth or sixth decade of life.[15,16] The sporadic ELST have no gender predilection, whereas tumors associated with VHL have a female preponderance of 2:1.[13]

Cochleovestibular dysfunction is the most common presenting symptom for ELST. Nearly all patients will have some degree of SNHL (86%–100%), which is often asymmetric and corresponds with tumor extension.[15–17] SNHL that presents as a sudden loss is likely from intralabyrinthine hemorrhage followed by inflammation and neural

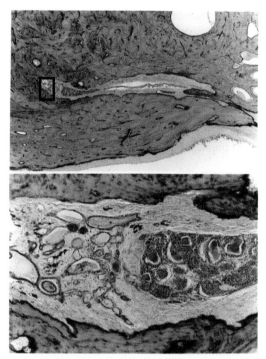

Fig. 1. Histopathologic specimen from the right temporal bone (contralateral to the gross tumor) of a patient with Von Hippel–Lindau (VHL) disease (case 1, autopsy). (*Top*) Epithelial proliferation is present in the endolymphatic sac (stain: hematoxylin and eosin [H&E]; original magnification, ×50). Black box highlights area of magnification bellow. (*Bottom*) Higher magnification demonstrates the papillary and follicular morphology of aggressive papillary adenomatous tumors of the endolymphatic sac (stain: H&E; original magnification, ×200). (*From* Megerian CA, McKenna MJ, Nuss RC, et al. Endolymphatic sac tumors: histologic confirmation, clinical characterization, and implication in von Hippel-Lindau disease. Laryngoscope 1995;105:803; with permission.)

degeneration. SNHL that has a more gradual progression is caused by either direct invasion of adjacent sensory structures within the otic capsule or the development of endolymphatic hydrops.[18–20] Tinnitus frequently accompanies the SNHL (71%–89%).

Vertigo and aural fullness are the next most common symptoms affecting 70% and 37% of patients, respectively.[16,20] As the ELST grows, it blocks endolymph reabsorption and may produce excess fluid, both of which create secondary hydrops. The combination of SNHL, tinnitus, aural fullness, and vertigo mimics Meniere disease and may delay diagnosis.[13,21,22] This point illustrates that Meniere disease is a diagnosis of exclusion and imaging to exclude lesions like ELST is a necessary part of the workup.[23]

Other cranial neuropathies may also be present with ELST, but are less common than the previously mentioned symptoms. Facial nerve weakness is seen 5% to 33% of cases.[16,20] Trigeminal nerve and glossopharyngeal nerve deficits have also been reported. The involvement of other cranial nerves depends on tumor extension, which proceeds along 4 common vectors.[13] From its origin at the posteromedial aspect of the temporal bone, ELST most commonly spread in a posterior direction to the cerebellopontine angle or posterior fossa. If large enough, brainstem compression may contribute to poor vestibular function and cause headache symptoms. Lateral extension via the middle ear and mastoid is the next most common pathway and may involve the facial nerve or produce symptoms that mimic chronic otitis media and Eustachian tube dysfunction.[24] ELST have even been diagnosed as masses in the external auditory canal. Superior extension through the semicircular canals and into the middle fossa can also contribute to imbalance. Finally, anterior extension along the petrous ridge may invade the clivus, cavernous sinus, or sphenoid sinus. Death has been reported secondary to intracranial extension and vascular compromise. There have been no reports of distant hematogenous metastasis, although "drop metastasis" to the spinal column causing lower extremity paralysis has been reported.[25,26]

IMAGING

Characteristic radiographic findings can help to diagnosis ELST and aid in preoperative planning. In 1997, Mukherji and colleagues[27] provided the first comprehensive radiologic review of ELST. Other reports have also added to the radiologic profile.[28–30]

CT shows enhancing soft tissue masses with bone erosion centered over the endolymphatic sac at the posteromedial temporal bone. Prominent intratumor (central) calcific spiculation and posterior rim calcification are often seen. An intralabyrinthine hyperdense signal on noncontrasted images may suggest an intralabyrinthine hemorrhage in radiographically small or undetectable tumors. On MRI, ELST show heterogenous foci of low and high signal intensity on T1-weighted and T2-weighted imaging. The hyperintense areas on noncontrast T1-weighted MRI is owing to intraparenchymal hemorrhage and subsequent deposition of methemoglobin, hemosiderin, and cholesterol crystals. The hypointense areas may reflect residual bone or prominent calcification. When given contrast, these tumors generally show heterogenous enhancement (**Fig. 2**).[29,30]

Angiography may aid in the diagnosis of ELST and may enable preoperative embolization. All ELST are hypervascular. The blood supply primarily arises from the external carotid artery system, although contributions from the internal carotid artery have also been described. The blood supply for the endolymphatic duct arises from either the inferior tympanic artery, a branch of the ascending pharyngeal artery, or the dural branch of the stylomastoid artery, a branch from the posterior auricular artery.[27] Even with these radiographic features, the ELST diagnosis can be challenging to distinguish from other lesions on the differential, such as paraganglioma (glomus jugulare or glomus tympanicum), choroid plexus tumor, metastasis, eosinophilic granuloma, meningioma, arachnoid granulation, aneurysmal bone cyst, or a primary bone tumor.[30,31]

VON HIPPEL–LINDAU DISEASE

VHL disease was first described in the early 20th century by the German ophthalmologist Eugene von Hippel and the Swedish pathologist Avrid Lindau.[32] VHL disease is an autosomal-dominant, multisystem disorder characterized by cerebellar hemangioblastomas, retinal angiomas, renal or pancreatic cysts, renal cell carcinoma, pheochromocytomas, and other visceral tumors. VHL disease has a prevalence of 1 in 39,000 individuals, of which 11% will develop ELST and, of those patients, 30% will have bilateral lesions.[33–35]

Since its identification in 1993, the genetics and molecular mechanism of tumorigenesis have been widely studied. The *VHL* locus at chromosome 3p25.5 encodes pVHL, a tumor suppressor that functions as an ubiquitin ligase targeting hypoxia inducible factor 1-alpha (HIF-1-alpha) for proteasomal degradation. In normal

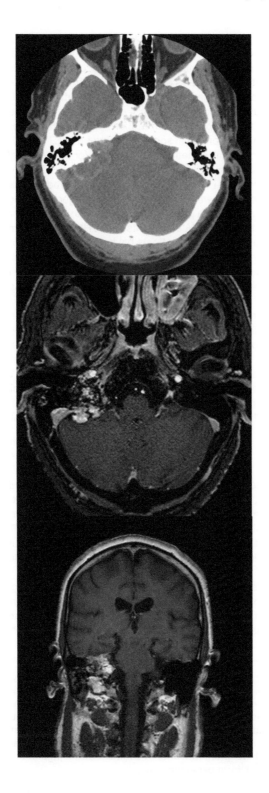

situations, patients have 2 copies of the wild-type (normal) *VHL* allele. Individuals with VHL disease inherit a mutated copy of the *VHL* allele. Then when a spontaneous mutation occurs in the other *VHL* allele, the patient becomes susceptible to VHL-related tumors. HIFs regulate angiogenesis and cell metabolism; thus, VHL-related tumors are often highly vascular.[36,37] Pharmacologic agents targeting HIF and its downstream targets remain investigational. There are 4 subtypes of VHL disease (types 1, 2A, 2B, and 2C) based on the type of *VHL* mutation. Although these subtypes can predict clinical disease manifestation, an association between ELST and VHL subtype has not yet been identified.[37,38] Still, genetic testing to look for a *VHL* mutation is recommended for all patients with an ELST.

Retrospective studies of ELST in VHL disease and sporadic cases highlight key differences. ELST associated with VHL present at a younger age (range, 7–63 years old; mean, 31.3) and have a female predominance (2:1 ratio). Microscopic tumor foci may explain the observation that 65% of patients with VHL disease demonstrate a degree of SNHL despite only 6% of those patients having detectable tumor on MRI. The slow tumor progression may also explain an average delay of 10 years between onset of symptoms and radiologic tumor detection. Aside from early disease onset, the cochleovestibular manifestations of ELST with or without VHL disease association are similar.[15,34,39]

Currently, there are no established international guidelines for surveillance and early detection of ELST. Institutional practices vary and may utilize audiometry and/or MRI to monitor disease progression in patients with known VHL disease.[38] The routine use of MRI every 12 to 36 months for surveillance of hemangioblastomas of the central nervous system has led to earlier ELST detection in patients with VHL disease. Early detection of ELST enables less morbid operations with a better chance of cure and hearing preservation. The prospect of hearing preservation is particularly important for patients with VHL disease who are at increased risk of bilateral ELST.[15,35]

HISTOLOGY

ELST are low-grade, locally infiltrative, highly vascular, poorly circumscribed neoplasms. They are grossly described as polypoid lesions. On light microscopy, they have 2 distinct patterns: papillary and follicular. The papillary pattern refers to cuboidal or low columnar epithelial cells arranged in papillary projections (**Fig. 3**). In contrast, the follicular pattern is cystic with spaces that contain proteinaceous material reminiscent of thyroid follicle, but thyroglobulin stains are negative. Some tumors may display both features.[5,13,18]

Cytologic features include homogenous cells with rare mitotic figures and no areas of necrosis. Light microscopy differentials include middle ear adenoma, adenocarcinoma, paraganglioma, choroid plexus papilloma, adenoid cystic carcinoma of ceruminal gland and metastatic adenocarcinoma (thyroid and kidney).[14,40]

Fig. 2. Radiographic findings in a patient with a right-sided endolymphatic sac tumor (ELST). (*Top*) This CT temporal bone without contrast demonstrates a lesion centered at the posterior aspect of the right petrous bone and demonstrates bony invasion as well as intratumor calcifications. (*Middle*) Axial T1-weighted MRI with contrast that shows heterogeneous enhancement. (*Bottom*) Coronal T1-weighted MRI with contrast that shows heterogeneous enhancement and extension through the jugular fossa. The "salt and pepper" appearance of the T1-weighted MRI and involvement of the jugular bulb can make it difficult to distinguish ELST from paraganglioma.

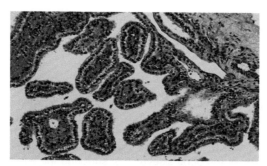

Fig. 3. Light microscopy of an endolymphatic sac tumor (ELST). Grossly, ESLT are described as highly vascular, polypoid lesions that are poorly circumscribed and may infiltrate into adjacent soft tissue or bone. Hematoxylin and eosin staining shows a papillary growth pattern with common cystic areas lined by cuboidal to low-columnar epithelial cells disposed in a fibrous stroma (original magnification ×50).

Immunohistochemical staining helps to differentiate ELST from some of the entities previously described. The endolymphatic sac is a neuroectodermal-derived structure; therefore, ELST are cytokeratin and vimentin positive and the majority will be S-100 positive. Differentiating from paraganglioma may be aided by the chromogranin-negative immunohistochemical profile of ELST. Choroid plexus tumors are distinctly transthyretin positive, whereas ELST are negative. ELST are thyroglobulin negative, a feature that helps to differentiate them from metastatic thyroid cancer.[14,15,40]

STAGING

In 2004, a retrospective analysis of 149 ELST led to an anatomic classification system, the Bambakidis and Megerian grading system for ELST.[15] This grading scheme also provides surgical treatment options based on the extent of tumor invasion and hearing status (**Table 1**).[41] The review by Bambakidis and colleagues demonstrated that ELST in patients with VHL disease tends to be diagnosed at a lower grade compared to sporadic cases (grade 1, 40% vs 25%; grade II, 50% vs 58%; grade III 8% vs 14%; grade IV, 2% vs 4%; $P<.05$). This lower grade at the time of diagnosis reflects an increased

Table 1		
Grading and treatment system for endolymphatic tumors		
Grade	**Tumor Extent**	**Surgical Options**
I	Confined to temporal bone, middle ear cavity, and/or external auditory canal	Hearing preservation with retrolabyrinthine transdural approach
II	Extension into posterior fossa	Extended retrolabyrinthine transdural approach, approach with labyrinthectomy if hearing is poor[a]
III	Extension in posterior fossa and middle cranial fossa	Subtemporal craniotomy with petrosectomy[a]
IV	Extension to clivus and/or sphenoid wing	Staged anterior and posterior fossa techniques[a]

[a] Preoperative embolization for grades II–IV and postoperative stereotactic radiosurgery for postoperative residual disease may be an adjunctive.

Adapted from Bambakidis NC, Megerian CA, Ratcheson RA. Differential grade of Endolymphatic Sac Tumor extension by virtue of von Hippel-Lindau disease status. Otol Neurotol 2004;25:773–81; with permission.

utilization of intracranial imaging, specifically MRI, for surveillance of patients with VHL disease. Whether the ELST is sporadic or VHL associated, early diagnosis and lower tumor grades offers greater potential for hearing preservation and cure.

TREATMENT

The mainstay of ELST management remains complete surgical excision. The evolution of operative approaches for the small ELST has paralleled our knowledge of the behavior and position of this tumor within the endolymphatic sac and substantial portions of the osseous endolymphatic duct. The most effective method that allows for removal of both sides of the dural sleeves that surround the endolymphatic sac has been called the retrolabyrinthine–transdural approach or the retrolabyrinthine posterior petrosectomy approach.[19,35]

For the retrolabyrinthine–transdural approach, the patient is placed supine, with their head turned away from the surgeon. Hair is shaved, but head pins are not necessary. A facial nerve monitor is used. Using an extended postauricular incision, a mastoidectomy is performed with identification of the horizontal semicircular canal and facial nerve. The jugular bulb is skeletonized, as is the tegmental dura and sinodural angle. After identifying and skeletonizing the posterior semicircular canal, the outline of a bulging tumor-filled endolymphatic sac is often seen (**Fig. 4**). The endolymphatic duct is then followed with a diamond drill behind the posterior semicircular canal toward the vestibule and tumor is carefully removed. If the posterior semicircular canal is violated, it can be sealed quickly with bone wax. A margin of at least 0.5 cm around the sac on healthy posterior fossa dura is obtained as the sac and duct are removed en bloc (**Figs. 5** and **6**). This procedure is performed after removing tumor-laden bone from the posterior dural surface using a high-speed drill. The antrum is then sealed with bone wax. Abdominal fat and dural substitute are used to seal the dura, often with the aid of a tissue sealant to prevent cerebrospinal fluid leaks (**Fig. 7**).

A transmastoid approach, which carries the shortcoming of leaving the posterior sleeve of dura intact and potentially providing a site for tumor recurrence, has been described (**Fig. 8**).[35] Similarly, a posterior fossa (retrosigmoid) approach leaves the

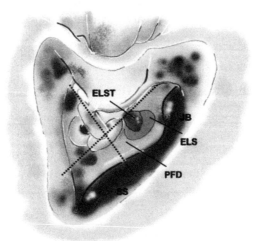

Fig. 4. Right mastoid cavity, demonstrating the endolymphatic sac (ELS), endolymphatic sac tumor (ELST), jugular bulb (JB), posterior fossa dura (PFD), and sigmoid sinus (SS). The dotted lines correspond with Donaldson's lines and the usual location of the ELS.

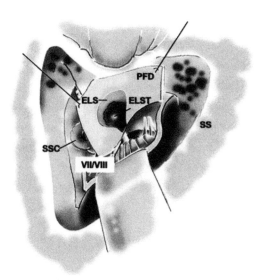

Fig. 5. Removal of an endolymphatic sac tumor (ELST) via a retrolabyrinthine–transdural approach, with elevation of the posterior fossa dura (PFD). Cranial nerves VII and VIII are seen in the cerebellopontine cistern. The semicircular canals are preserved. ELS, endolymphatic sac; SS, sigmoid sinus; SSC, superior semicircular canal.

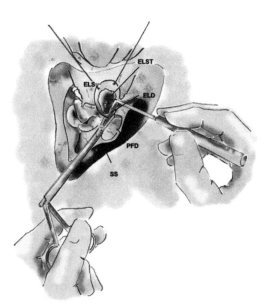

Fig. 6. Transmastoid removal of an endolymphatic sac tumor (ELST) from the right ear. The endolymphatic sac (ELS) has been elevated and retracted superiorly, exposing the ELST and preserving the posterior fossa dura (PFD). Excision of the lesion can be performed without violating the dura. ELD, endolymphatic duct; SS, sigmoid sinus.

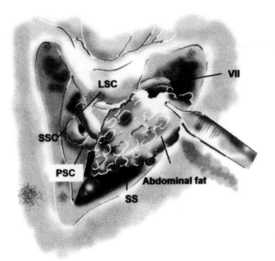

Fig. 7. After resection of a grade 1 endolymphatic sac tumor (ELST), the mastoid cavity is obliterated with abdominal fat. LSC, lateral semicircular canal; PSC, posterior semicircular canal; SS, sigmoid sinus; SSC, superior semicircular canal; VII, vertical portion of facial nerve.

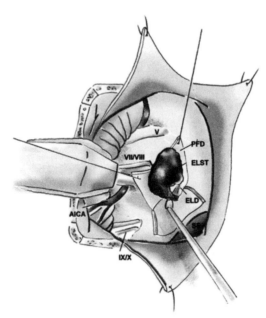

Fig. 8. Cerebellopontine angle as seen during a retrosigmoid craniotomy for removal of an endolymphatic sac tumor (ELST). The cerebellum is retracted medially. The endolymphatic sac (ELS) is seen halfway between the sigmoid sinus (SS) and internal auditory canal. The ELST is seen bulging into the posterior fossa. Once dura over the ELST has been opened and retracted, the tumor can be dissected from the sac and duct. This approach preserves hearing only if the contents of the labyrinth are not violated. PFD, posterior fossa dura.

anterior dural sleeve and does not afford visualization of the posterior semicircular canal during dissection of the endolymphatic duct.[19,35] Patients with poor or unserviceable hearing often have labyrinthine invasion; thus, a concomitant translabyrinthine approach is required.

Larger grade II lesions with their increased vascularity and posterior fossa invasion are at risk for a significant amount of intraoperative bleeding. For these tumors, preoperative embolization is advised. Based on the size of the lesion and middle fossa extension, a subtemporal transpetrous approach may be required. These approaches typically provide very good tumor control.

The House Clinic recently published one of the largest single institutional experiences with surgical management of ELST.[16] They reported 18 patients, all treated with microsurgical techniques for tumors with a mean size of 2.4 cm. Total resection was possible in 17 of 18 tumors (94%), and after a mean follow-up of 67 months, 16 patients (89%) remained disease free. Consistent with the literature, the majority of patients (89%) presented with SNHL. The 2 patients with serviceable preoperative hearing both maintained serviceable hearing after their retrolabyrinthine–transdural approach. Good preoperative facial function, graded as a House-Brackmann II or better, was present in 13 of 18 patients (72%) and all but 2 of them maintained good facial function. Excluding cranial nerve VII and VIII injuries, the most common complication was new onset of other cranial neuropathies (cranial nerves IX, X, or XII) in 4 of 18 patients (22%). Additionally, there were 3 cerebrospinal fluid leaks and 2 cases of hydrocephalus. Friedman and colleagues[16] also reviewed the ELST literature and found a 26% surgical complication rate.

Other authors have reported good oncologic outcomes using microsurgical techniques for ELST. For instance, Heffner[5] in 1989 reported 11 of 16 patients (69%) with no evidence of disease (NED) after a mean follow-up of 61 months. Luff and colleagues[42] in 2002 reported 3 of 3 patients (100%) with NED after a mean follow-up of 60 months. Rodrigues and colleagues[43] in 2004 reported 6 of 7 patients (86%) with NED after a mean follow-up of 69 months. Doherty and colleagues[44] in 2007 reported 3 of patients 3 (100%) with NED after a mean follow-up of 32 months. Bae and colleagues[45] in 2008 reported 3 of 4 patients (75%) with NED after a mean follow-up of 33 months. Kim and colleagues[39] in 2012 reported 30 of 33 tumors (91%) in 31 consecutive patients with NED after a mean follow-up of 50 months. Carlson and colleagues[46] in 2013 reported 10 of 11 patients (91%) who had primary ELST treated with microsurgery being NED after a mean follow-up of 63 months. In total, disease was eradicated with the microsurgical techniques in 82 of 95 patients (86%).

The role of radiation therapy for the management of ELST remains controversial. Currently, stereotactic radiotherapy with Gamma knife can be used in patients with unresectable disease, subtotal resections, or patients not deemed surgical candidates.[13,39,46] There are no data to support a therapeutic role for chemotherapy in the management of ELST.

The best approach to preserve hearing in grade I ELST remains to be determined. The translabyrinthine approach is advantageous for good visualization of the posterior semicircular canal, thus preventing inadvertent violation of the labyrinth. To resect both dural leaflets of the endolymphatic sac, Megerian and colleagues[35] recommended the retrolabyrinthine–transdural approach because it enables excellent visualization of the labyrinthine structures as well as visualization of the posterior petrous bone. The drawback of the retrolabyrinthine–transdural approach is the need to repair the dura with abdominal fat or other mechanisms. All 3 of these techniques have been described for successful hearing preservation.[16,35,47] In rare cases of bilateral deafness after resection in patients who have VHL, cochlear implantation remains a viable option for hearing rehabilitation.[48,49]

SUMMARY

The ELST is a slow-growing, locally aggressive neoplasm that originates from the epithelium of the endolymphatic sac and duct. Disease progression can lead to profound SNHL, posterior fossa invasion, brainstem compression, drop metastasis, and eventual death. Early diagnosis and surgical attention are the primary objectives in the management of patients who have ELST. The association between ELST and VHL disease has increased our knowledge of this rare tumor. This article describes the latest rationale and techniques for hearing preservation surgery and a review of the latest developments surrounding this disease entity.

ACKNOWLEDGMENTS

The authors thank Dr George B. Wanna (Department of Otolaryngology-Head and Neck Surgery, Vanderbilt University) for providing the images used in **Fig. 2**.

REFERENCES

1. Johnstone JM, Lennox B, Watson AJ. Five cases of hidradenoma of the external auditory meatus: so-called ceruminoma. J Pathol Bacteriol 1957;73:421–7.
2. Harrison K, Cronin J, Greenwood N. Ceruminous adenocarcinoma arising in the middle ear. J Laryngol Otol 1974;88:363–8.
3. Hyams VJ, Michaels L. Benign adenomatous neoplasm (adenoma) of the middle ear. Clin Otolaryngol 1976;1:17–26.
4. Gaffey MJ, Mills SE, Fechner RE, et al. Aggressive papillary middle ear tumor: a clinicopathologic entity distinct from middle ear adenoma. Am J Surg Pathol 1988;12:790–7.
5. Heffner DK. Low-grade adenocarcinoma of probable endolymphatic sac origin: a clinicopathologic study of 20 cases. Cancer 1989;64:2292–302.
6. Hassard AD, Boudreau SF, Cron CC. Adenoma of the endolymphatic sac. J Otolaryngol 1984;12:213–6.
7. Li JC, Brackmann DE, Lo WW, et al. Reclassification of aggressive adenomatous mastoid neoplasms as endolymphatic sac tumors. Laryngoscope 1993;103: 1342–8.
8. Castleman B, McNeely BU. Case records of the Massachusetts General Hospital: case 47-1966. N Engl J Med 1966;275:950–9.
9. Naguib MG, Chou SN, Mastri A. Radiation therapy of a choroid plexus papilloma of the cerebellopontine angle with bone involvement. J Neurosurg 1981;54: 245–7.
10. Blamires TL, Friedmann I, Moffat DA. Von Hippel Lindau disease associated with an invasive choroid plexus tumor presenting as a middle ear mass. J Laryngol Otol 1992;106:429–35.
11. Poe DS, Tarlov EC, Thomas CB, et al. Aggressive papillary tumors of the temporal bone. Otolaryngol Head Neck Surg 1993;108:80–6.
12. Pollak A, Bohmer A, Spycher M, et al. Are papillary adenomas endolymphatic sac tumors? Ann Otol Rhinol Laryngol 1995;104:613–9.
13. Megerian CA, McKenna MJ, Nuss RC, et al. Endolymphatic sac tumors: histologic confirmation, clinical characterization, and implication in von Hippel-Lindau disease. Laryngoscope 1995;105:801–8.
14. Megerian CA, Pilch BZ, Bahn A, et al. Differential expression of transthyretin in papillary tumors of the endolymphatic sac and choroid plexus. Laryngoscope 1997;107:216–21.

15. Bambakidis NC, Megerian CA, Ratcheson RA. Differential grading of endolymphatic sac tumor extension by virtue of von Hippel-Lindau disease status. Otol Neurotol 2004;25(5):773–81.
16. Friedman RA, Hoa M, Brackmann DE. Surgical management of endolymphatic sac tumors. J Neurol Surg B 2013;74:12–9.
17. Hansen MR, Luxford WM. Surgical outcomes in patients with endolymphatic sac tumors. Laryngoscope 2004;114:1470–4.
18. Lonser RR, Kim HF, Butman JA, et al. Tumors of the endolymphatic sac in von Hippel-Lindau disease. N Engl J Med 2004;350:2481–6.
19. Kim HF, Butman JA, Brewer C, et al. Tumors of the endolymphatic sac in patients with von Hippel-Lindau disease: implications for their natural history, diagnosis, and treatment. J Neurosurg 2005;102:503–12.
20. Butman JA, Kim HF, Baggenstos M, et al. Mechanism of morbid hearing loss associated with tumors of the endolymphatic sac in von Hippel-Lindau disease. JAMA 2007;298(1):41–8.
21. Ong YK, Chee NW, Hwang PY, et al. Endolymphatic sac tumour: a rare cause of recurrent vertigo. Singapore Med J 2006;47(7):627–30.
22. Raghunandhan S, Vijaya Krishnan P, Murali S, et al. Endolymphatic sac tumour: a neoplastic cause for Meniere's syndrome. Indian J Otolaryngol Head Neck Surg 2014;66(S1):S352–5.
23. Committee on Hearing and Equilibrium guidelines for the diagnosis and evaluation of therapy in Meniere's disease. Otolaryngol Head Neck Surg 1995;13:181–5.
24. Mishra G, Sharma Y, Padhya C, et al. Endolymphatic duct papillary tumour: captured undercover of complicated chronic otitis media. Indian J Otolaryngol Head Neck Surg 2013;65(Suppl 3):S662–4.
25. Bambakidis NC, Rodrique T, Megerian CA, et al. Endolymphatic sac tumor metastasis to the spine: case report. J Neurosurg Spine 2005;3:68–70.
26. Tay KY, Yu E, Kassel E. Spinal metastasis from endolymphatic sac tumor. AJNR Am J Neuroradiol 2007;28:613–4.
27. Mukherji SK, Albernaz VS, Lo WW, et al. Papillary endolymphatic sac tumors: CT, MR imaging and angiographic findings in 20 patients. Radiology 1997;202: 801–8.
28. Lo WW, Applegate LJ, Carberry JN, et al. Endolymphatic sac tumors: radiologic appearance. Radiology 1993;189:199–204.
29. Mukherji SK, Castillo M. Adenocarcinoma of the endolymphatic sac: imaging features and preoperative embolization. Neuroradiology 1996;38:179–80.
30. Patel N, Wiggins RH, Shelton C. The radiologic diagnosis of endolymphatic sac tumors. Laryngoscope 2006;116:40–6.
31. Alkonyi B, Gunthner-Lengsfeld T, Rak K, et al. An endolymphatic sac tumor with imaging features of aneurysmal bone cysts: differential diagnosis considerations. Childs Nerv Syst 2014;30(9):1583–8.
32. Bamps S, Van Calenbergh F, De Vleeschouwer S, et al. What the neurosurgeon should know about hemangioblastoma, both sporadic and in von Hippel-Lindau disease: a literature review. Surg Neurol Int 2013;4:145–54.
33. Neumann HP, Wiestler OD. Clustering of features of von Hippel-Lindau syndrome: evidence for a complex genetic locus. Lancet 1991;337:1052–4.
34. Manski TJ, Heffner DK, Glenn GM, et al. Endolymphatic sac tumors: a source of morbid hearing loss in von Hippel-Lindau disease. JAMA 1997;277(18):1461–6.
35. Megerian CA, Haynes DS, Poe DS, et al. Hearing preservation surgery for small endolymphatic sac tumors in patients with von Hippel-Lindau syndrome. Otol Neurotol 2002;23:378–87.

36. Kawahara N, Kume H, Ueki K, et al. VHL gene inactivation in endolymphatic sac tumor associated with von Hippel-Lindau disease. Neurology 1999;53:208–10.

37. Kaelin WG. Molecular basis of the VHL hereditary cancer syndrome. Nat Rev Cancer 2002;2:673–82.

38. Poulsen ML, Gimsing S, Kosteljanetz M, et al. von Hippel-Lindau disease: surveillance strategy for endolymphatic sac tumors. Genet Med 2011;13(12):1032–41.

39. Kim HJ, Hagan M, Butman JA, et al. Surgical resection of endolymphatic sac tumors in von Hippel-Lindau disease: findings, results, and indications. Laryngoscope 2012;123:477–83.

40. Devaney KO, Ferlito A, Rinaldo A. Endolymphatic sac tumor (low-grade papillary adenocarcinoma) of the temporal bone. Acta Otolaryngol 2003;123(9):1022–6.

41. Megerian CA, Semaan MT. Evaluation and management of endolymphatic sac and duct tumors. Otolaryngol Clin North Am 2007;40:463–78.

42. Luff DA, Simmons M, Malik T, et al. Endolymphatic sac tumours. J Laryngol Otol 2002;116:398–401.

43. Rodrigues S, Fagan P, Turner J. Endolymphatic sac tumors: a review of the St. Vincent's hospital experience. Otol Neurotol 2004;25:599–603.

44. Doherty JK, Yong M, Maceri D. Endolymphatic sac tumor: a report of 3 cases and discussion of management. Ear Nose Throat J 2007;86:30–5.

45. Bae CW, Cho YH, Chung JW, et al. Endolymphatic sac tumors: report of four cases. J Korean Neurosurg Soc 2008;44:268–72.

46. Carlson ML, Thom JJ, Driscoll CL, et al. Management of primary and recurrent endolymphatic sac tumors. Otol Neurotol 2013;34:939–43.

47. Schipper J, Maier W, Rosahl SK, et al. Endolymphatic sac tumors: surgical management. J Otolaryngol 2006;35(6):387–94.

48. Belal A. Is cochlear implantation possible after acoustic tumor removal? Otol Neurotol 2001;22:497–500.

49. Boccio CM, Raffo GM, Parsini C. Cochlear implantation in a bilateral endolymphatic sac tumor patient. A case report. Int J Pediatr Otorhinolaryngol 2007;71:1803–7.

Contemporary Management of Jugular Paragangliomas

George B. Wanna, MD[a],*, Alex D. Sweeney, MD[a],
David S. Haynes, MD[a], Matthew L. Carlson, MD[b]

KEYWORDS

- Jugular paraganglioma • Cranial nerves • Glomus tumor • Jugular foramen
- Carotid artery

KEY POINTS

- Jugular paragangliomas are the most common tumors of the jugular foramen.
- The management of jugular paragangliomas is challenging because of their close proximity to cranial nerves (CN) and the internal carotid artery.
- Surgery, radiation, and observation are all viable management options and should be individualized to the patient.
- At the authors' center, there has been a paradigm shift toward conservatism in selected cases in order to minimize morbidity.

INTRODUCTION

Jugular paragangliomas (JPs) are the most common primary neoplasms of the jugular foramen, arising from the paraganglion cells within the adventitia of the jugular bulb. They are slow-growing, highly vascularized tumors that are usually diagnosed during the fourth to fifth decades of life, affecting women 3 times more frequently than men. Although considered histologically benign, the management of jugular paragangliomas is challenging because of their infiltrative nature and close proximity to the facial nerve and lower cranial nerves (CN), carotid canal, posterior fossa meninges, and otic capsule.[1–4] Historically, gross total microsurgical resection was considered the

Financial Material & Support: No funding or other support was required for this study.
Conflict(s) of Interest to Declare: There are no relevant conflicts of interest to disclose.
[a] Department of Otolaryngology–Head and Neck Surgery, Vanderbilt University, 7209 Medical Center East, South Tower, 1215 21st Avenue South, Nashville, TN 37232, USA; [b] Department of Otolaryngology–Head and Neck Surgery, Mayo Clinic School of Medicine, 200 1st Street Southwest, Rochester, MN 55905, USA
* Corresponding author. Department of Otolaryngology–Head and Neck Surgery, The Bill Wilkerson Center for Otolaryngology & Communication Sciences, 7209 Medical Center East, South Tower, 1215 21st Avenue South, Nashville, TN 37232-8605.
E-mail address: george.wanna@vanderbilt.edu

Otolaryngol Clin N Am 48 (2015) 331–341
http://dx.doi.org/10.1016/j.otc.2014.12.007
0030-6665/15/$ – see front matter © 2015 Elsevier Inc. All rights reserved.

Abbreviations	
CN	Cranial nerves
GJT	Glomus jugulare tumor
JP	Jugular paragangliomas

treatment of choice, offering complete eradication of disease; however, this strategy may cause significant morbidity, even in the hands of experienced surgeons.[5]

In an effort to explore less invasive treatment methods, stereotactic radiosurgery began gaining popularity in the early 1990s, and today has become the primary treatment modality of choice for many centers. The primary benefit of radiation therapy is a lower risk of up-front cranial neuropathy compared with gross total resection; however, tumor control and length of follow-up in these studies are variable.[6,7]

More recently, observation has been considered for select patients such as those with small tumors and few attributable symptoms, those with multicentric disease and contralateral lower cranial neuropathy, or elderly and infirm patients without brainstem compression. The data concerning observation for JP are scarce, and few centers have looked into the clinical course of untreated JP.[8,9] Such data are needed in order to compare against outcomes with radiation therapy. For example, if it was demonstrated that a large number of tumors do not grow for extended periods of observation, it could be argued that radiation therapy should be reserved until there is definitive evidence of growth.

The Otology Group of Vanderbilt has over 40 years of experience with JP. In the authors' practice, most tumors are managed with microsurgery; however, over the last decade, the authors' group has adopted a less aggressive approach in select patients in order to minimize cranial nerve morbidity. In this article, the authors report their experience managing JP, highlighting the paradigm shift in treatment at the authors' center.

DISEASE PRESENTATION

Pulsatile tinnitus is the most common presenting symptom in patients with JP, followed by hearing decline.[10] Hearing loss is usually conductive in nature but can be sensorineural or mixed.[11] Lower cranial neuropathies resulting in dysphagia, hoarseness, shoulder weakness, and tongue hemiparesis are less common and are usually seen with larger tumors that extend through the medial wall of the jugular bulb. Headache and vomiting are usually late signs associated with increased intracranial pressure caused by brainstem compression and fourth ventricle effacement.[12]

A pulsatile red middle ear mass behind an intact tympanic membrane is the most common finding on physical examination (**Fig. 1**). By definition, a glomus jugulare extends from the jugular bulb and hypotympanum into the middle ear space. Therefore, the middle ear component only represents the tip of the iceberg. Although not universally present, increased canal and tympanic membrane vascularity surrounding the inferiorly based middle red ear mass may result in the characteristic, rising sun appearance. Less commonly, the tympanic portion of the tumor may erupt into the ear canal, resulting in bloody otorrhea.

In contrast to visceral paragangliomas, head and neck paragangliomas are rarely (<4%) secretory.[13] Patients reporting a history of palpitations, sweats, flushing, syncope, hypertension, and headaches should be screened for serum and urine catecholamine levels. If elevated catecholamine levels are found, the patient should undergo further imaging to rule out pheochromocytoma or multicentric paraganglioma disease.

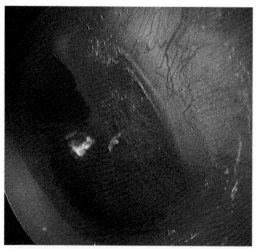

Fig. 1. Otoscopic examination demonstrating a red mass behind an intact tympanic membrane.

IMAGING

A careful review of fine-cut temporal bone computed tomography (CT) and MRI with gadolinium is critical to differentiating jugular foramen tumors. The most common lesions to involve the jugular foramen are JP, meningiomas (**Fig. 2**), and lower cranial nerve schwannomas (**Fig. 3**). Metastatic disease and endolymphatic sac tumors may also secondarily involve this region (**Fig. 4**). On CT and MRI, JPs demonstrate a diffusely infiltrative pattern of disease resulting in bony destruction and early erosion of the jugulo–carotid spine (**Fig. 5**). Vascular flow voids within the tumor result in a characteristic salt-and-pepper appearance on T1 and T2 weighted MRI, and the tumor avidly enhances with contrast administration (**Fig. 6**). Although not completely reliable, most JPs demonstrate middle ear extension, while meningiomas and schwannomas rarely do so. In contrast, meningiomas commonly demonstrate dural tails with en plaque growth and are often associated with underlying hyperostosis. Finally, schwannomas often "dumbbell" between the neck and posterior fossa, with a bottle neck at the jugular foramen. CT generally reveals a widened sharply demarcated jugular foramen without bony destruction.[14,15]

TUMOR CLASSIFICATION

Multiple proposed classifications have been used, and none has gained universal acceptance. Tumor classifications described by Fisch and Glasscock and Jackson are the most commonly used.[16–18]

GENETIC SCREENING

Familial head and neck paragangliomas are associated with germline mutations in genes encoding subunits of succinate dehydrogenase (SDH), which plays a role in the Krebs cycle. Though genetic evaluation of patients with head and neck paragangliomas is emerging as an important topic in the diagnosis and management of these tumors, the most cost-effective way of screening at-risk patients is not yet clear. Because 30% of sporadic head and neck paragangliomas are caused by germline

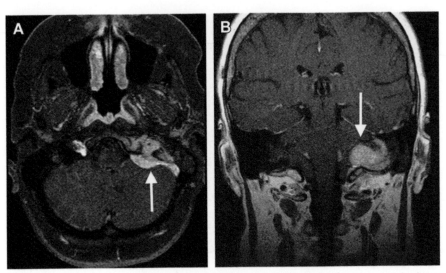

Fig. 2. (*A*) Axial cut of a T1 MRI with contrast showing a left jugular foramen meningioma. The tumor is designated by the white arrow. (*B*) Coronal cut of a T1 MRI with contrast showing a left jugular foramen meningioma. The tumor is designated by the white arrow.

mutation, Bodeker and colleagues recommend molecular genetic screening for SDHB, SDHC, and SDHD in all head and neck paragangliomas.[19,20] The authors' practice has been to offer patients genetic counseling and to collect and bank deidentified blood and tumor DNA from patients with JP undergoing surgery for future studies.

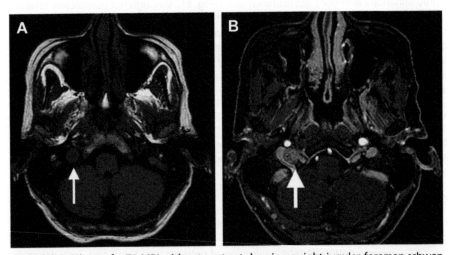

Fig. 3. (*A*) Axial cut of a T1 MRI without contrast showing a right jugular foramen schwannoma. The tumor is designated by the white arrow. (*B*) Axial cut of a T1 MRI with contrast showing enhancement of a right jugular foramen schwannoma. The tumor is designated by the white arrow.

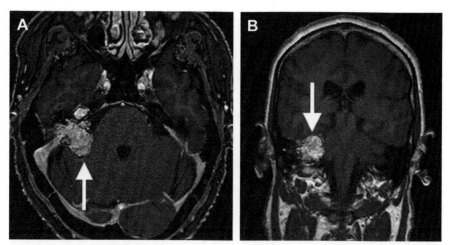

Fig. 4. (*A*) Axial cut T1 MRI with contrast showing a left endolymphatic sac tumor. The tumor is designated by the white arrow. (*B*) Coronal cut T1 MRI with contrast showing a left endolymphatic sac tumor. The tumor is designated by the white arrow.

MANAGEMENT
Embolization

Techniques of preoperative, transfermoral angiography with superselective embolization of feeding vessels have improved dramatically. Preoperative embolization may result in less intraoperative blood loss, thereby improving visualization, reducing morbidity, and increasing the probability of complete resection. Preoperative embolization is generally performed 24 to 72 hours before surgery. The authors' center most commonly uses Onyx (Covidien, Ireland), a nonadhesive liquid embolic agent. The authors' experience, thus far, is encouraging that the degree of embolization achievable with Onyx may decrease the need for intraoperative blood transfusion relative to other

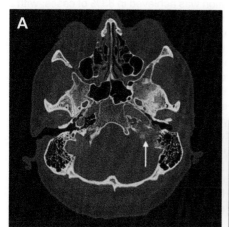
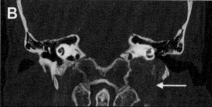

Fig. 5. High-resolution CT demonstrating the expected growth pattern of a GJT relative to the bone of the lateral skull base. The white arrow designates an area of tumor-associated bony destruction. (*A*) is an axial cut; (*B*) is a coronal cut.

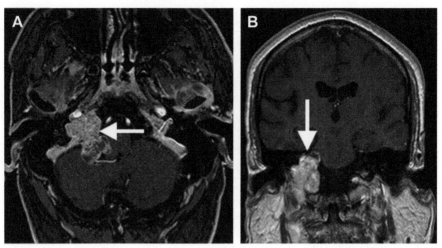

Fig. 6. Glomus jugulare as seen on a contrast-enhanced MRI scan. The arrow designates the tumor with a characteristic salt-and-pepper appearance. (*A*) is an axial cut; (*B*) is a coronal cut.

available substrates (**Fig. 7**). However, it is important to note that cranial nerve palsy can occur after embolization utilizing liquid and small particle agents such as Onyx.[19] Thus, preoperative patient counseling regarding the potential risks and benefits of embolization is warranted. Furthermore, a careful preoperative cranial nerve examination after embolization and immediately before surgery should be performed.

Surgery

Historically, microsurgery with gross total resection was considered the treatment strategy of choice for JP. Although gross total resection is possible in the majority of cases, it may result in debilitating cranial neuropathy and less commonly, vascular injury. In a study done by Sanna and colleagues,[21] 53 patients with Fisch class C or D JP were treated surgically. Gross total resection was achieved in 83% of cases, with a 10% tumor recurrence rate. The presence of new cranial neuropathy varied depending on the presence of intracranial extension, but was as high as 39%. Recently, the same group retrospectively reviewed 122 class C or D tumors. Gross tumor control was achieved in 86% of JPs, though 54% of the patients developed a postoperative lower cranial nerve injury. Cranial nerve IX was most commonly affected at last follow-up.[22] In another study including 119 patients, nearly 75% of patients had tumor control with surgical management, and new cranial neuropathies were noted in approximately 50% of patients after surgery.[23] Lastly, Fayad and colleagues,[3] examined the House Ear Clinic experience with glomus jugulare tumors (GJT), reporting total tumor removal in 81% of surgical cases. In this series, the incidence of postoperative cranial neuropathy varied according to tumor size. For patients with Fisch classification C4 and lower, the incidence of new cranial nerve injury varied from 8.7% to 13%, whereas for patients with classification of C4 and higher, the deficit ranged from 63.6% to 81.8%. Overall, 26.5% of patients in this series developed tumor recurrence at an average of 26 months.

In an effort to minimize morbidity and improve symptoms associated with disease, subtotal resection has been used with increasing frequency by many centers. Subtotal resection may be particularly relevant to older or infirm patients with advanced disease

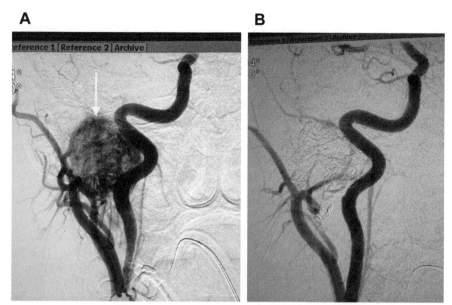

Fig. 7. Pre- and postembolization angiography of a GJT. (*A*) Pre-embolization image in which an arrow designates the highly vascularized tumor. (*B*) Postembolization image in which the major vascular pedicles for the tumor have been obliterated.

or younger patients with large tumors and intact CN who are troubled by aural symptoms such as pulsatile tinnitus, conductive hearing loss, and fullness. In a previous report, Cosetti and colleagues[9] reviewed the role of conservative management of JP and glomus tympanicum in patients over the age of 60 years. In a small sample, they found that 1 of 3 patients experienced tumor growth following subtotal resection nearly 6 years after treatment. In a study of patients over the age of 60 with advanced tumors, Willen and colleagues[24] identified no significant treatment failures at 19 months of mean follow-up with planned subtotal resection and adjuvant radiotherapy. Unfortunately, the published follow-up for these reports is generally short and limited by a relatively small number of cases. However, at this time, the authors' treatment algorithm has evolved to include subtotal resection. Akin to other benign skull base tumors, the authors believe that tumor recurrence is likely related to extent of resection. That is, the more tumor that is removed, the less likely the residual tumor is to grow.

Radiation

Because of the complexity of JP surgery, particularly regarding the close proximity of a vascular tumor to the facial nerve, the lower CN, and the carotid artery, nonsurgical management options such have radiation have emerged. Initially, fractionated external beam radiation was introduced for primary and salvage therapy. Control rates between 86% and 100% were described in early studies, which helped to establish the legitimacy of radiotherapy in the management algorithm for JP.[25–27] Over time, the use of therapeutic radiation evolved to employ stereotactic techniques that offer comparable tumor doses with less radiation injury to surrounding tissue.

Radiosurgery is now a well-accepted treatment modality for GJT. The treatment-specific tumor control and adverse effect profile has been shown to be least comparable to what can be achieved surgically. In a recent multicenter study of 132 patients, 18% with Jackson-Glasscock grade 4 tumors, Gamma Knife achieved tumor control in 93% of cases.[28] A meta-analysis evaluating 869 patients with glomus jugulare also lent credence to the utility of radiosurgery for JP.[29] Patients were divided in 4 groups: gross total resection, subtotal resection, subtotal resection followed by radiosurgery, and radiosurgery alone. Although differences in tumor size between the groups were not controlled, the authors found that the radiosurgery alone group had the best rates of tumor control and that gross total resection did not appear to offer significantly improved tumor control versus subtotal resection or subtotal resection followed by radiosurgery. Also noteworthy was the finding that patients who underwent gross total resection had significantly worse post-treatment cranial neuropathies when compared with patients undergoing radiosurgery. Although the optimal radiation regimen for JP tumors is not yet standardized,[30] the use of radiotherapy appears to be a valuable addition to the available therapeutic options.

Observation

The natural history of JP tumors is not well established, but evaluations of the wait-and-scan observation strategy have revealed that intervention may not always be necessary. In 1992, Van der Mey and colleagues[31] were among the first groups to provide evidence to this effect. In a subsequent report on 11 patients from the same center, it was revealed that 55% of tumors demonstrated radiologic progression, with a median growth rate of 0.8 mm per year.[8] A complicating factor in these series is the possibility that some of the observed tumors were glomus tympanicum rather than jugulare. However, other reports specific to glomus jugulare have since validated these findings. Recently, Prasad and colleagues[32] analyzed the outcomes of 23 Fisch type C and D tumors that were observed for a minimum of 3 years. They demonstrated that 65% of tumors remained stable or even regressed in size over a median follow-up of 61 months. To date this remains one of the largest series on the natural history of JP. The relative paucity of data on tumor observation can be attributed to the rarity of the tumor and historical trends toward intervention after diagnosis. However, although many tumors will potentially grow if left untreated,[7] the slow rate of growth for most tumors and potential complications of intervention make a wait-and-scan policy a worthy consideration after diagnosis.

THE OTOLOGY GROUP OF VANDERBILT EXPERIENCE

The Otology Group of Vanderbilt has been fortunate to be a tertiary referral center for JP tumors over the course of its existence. During this time, the management algorithm for these tumors has evolved to include tumor observation and planned subtotal resection, as well as gross total resection and radiation. A compilation of the authors' experience is described.

Surgery

Gross total resection
The Otology Group of Vanderbilt reported previously on 202 jugular paragangliomas treated over a period of 35 years. Total resection was achieved in 90% of cases, with a tumor recurrence rate of 6%. Preoperative cranial neuropathies were seen in 47% of cases, most commonly IX, X, and XII. New postoperative cranial nerve injuries were seen in 60% of patients, most commonly IX followed by XI, X, and XII. Nearly 12% (11.8%) of patients experienced disease recurrence requiring revision surgery. Total resection was possible in 93% of the cases involving recurrence, and 95% of

these patients experienced new postoperative cranial nerve deficits. Similar to what was seen in patients undergoing primary surgery, cranial nerve IX (77%) was the most commonly injured nerve.[5]

Subtotal resection

Subtotal resection of JP has become a mainstay of tumor management in the authors' practice. This technique has previously been described as applicable to select patients. Jackson and colleagues[33] published their experience using subtotal resection for attempted hearing preservation and noted that success in this regard was inversely related to tumor size. Over time, the authors' utilization of planned, subtotal resection has increased, particularly in younger patients with advanced tumors (Glasscock-Jackson grade 3–4) and functional lower CN. Reviewing the authors' experience from 1999 to 2013, 12 patients were identified from this demographic who underwent a planned subtotal resection. Although varying degrees of resection were identified on postoperative radiographic evaluation, no patient developed a permanent, postoperative cranial neuropathy, and no patient with a residual disease burden of less than 20% of the original tumor size experienced postoperative tumor growth at a mean of approximately 45 months of follow-up.[34] Although these results have helped to validate the authors' continued use of this strategy, the small size of the patient population and the relatively short time of follow-up prohibit a definitive conclusion that this technique is preferred in all cases. However, the authors believe that the general concept of cranial nerve- and carotid artery-sparing surgery is valid and should be considered in future clinical and research efforts.

Observation

As previously mentioned, the role of tumor observation remains unclear at this time. The authors recently reviewed their experience with tumor observation, focusing on patients with primary GJT and greater than 2 years of documented follow-up. Fifteen patients (80% female, mean age 64.2 years) with 16 tumors were evaluated. Patients were selected for tumor observation due to advanced age (73%) and patient preference (73%). Approximately 40% of tumors demonstrated growth at an average of 0.9 mm per year. However, no significant change in cranial nerve function was seen for most patients through nearly 7 years of follow-up. No deaths were attributable to tumor progression.[35] This experience has led the authors to consider observation with a wait-and-scan policy for patients who do not have brainstem compression or concern for malignancy.

Radiation

Over the last 10 years, 18 patients were treated with linear accelerator-based stereotactic radiotherapy for glomus jugulare at the authors' institution. Over 64% (64.3%) of patients underwent fractionated therapy, and the median follow-up was 28.8 months (range 18.6–56.1 months). Consistent with previous reports, fewer than 10% of patients had experienced disease progression at their last recorded MRI. Although the authors' experience is limited by a smaller patient sample size and relatively short follow-up, stereotactic radiotherapy currently remains an important part of the treatment algorithm.

SUMMARY

JPs continue to represent a management challenge. Surgical resection is complicated by the vascular nature of the tumor and its location relative to the lower CN, the facial nerve, and the carotid artery. Radiation has gained momentum as a viable strategy for tumor control, but this modality is not without adverse effects, and the natural history of many tumors may involve a lack of significant growth and symptom progression. Cranial nerve- and carotid-sparing subtotal resection may prove to be a valuable strategy in experienced hands, as may hybrid techniques that incorporate initial observation, subtotal resection, and adjuvant radiation. The role of genomic sequencing, both patient- and tumor-based, may also become a significant adjunct to tumor therapy, as this technology becomes readily available and cost-effective.

REFERENCES

1. Gulya A. The glomus tumor and its biology. Laryngoscope 1993;103(11 Suppl 60):7–15.
2. Jackson C. Glomus tympanicum and glomus jugulare tumors. Otolaryngol Clin North Am 2001;34(5):941–70.
3. Fayad JN, Bahar K, Brackmann DE. Jugular foramen tumors: clinical characteristics and treatment outcomes. Otol Neurotol 2010;31(2):299–305.
4. Jackson C. Basic surgical principles of neurotologic skull base surgery. Laryngoscope 1993;103(Suppl 60):29–44.
5. Kaylie D, O'Malley M, Auline J, et al. Neurotologic surgery for glomus tumors. Otolaryngol Clin North Am 2007;40:625–49.
6. Foote R, Pollack B, Gorman D, et al. Glomus jugulare tumor: tumor control and complications after stereotactic radiosurgery. Head Neck 2002;24(4):332–9.
7. Pollock B. Stereotactic radiosurgery in patients with glomus jugulare tumors. Neurosurg Focus 2004;17(2):E10.
8. Jansen JC, van den Berg R, Kuiper A, et al. Estimation of growth rate in patients with head and neck paragangliomas influences the treatment proposal. Cancer 2000;88:2811–6.
9. Cosetti M, Linstrom C, Alexiades G, et al. Glomus tumors in patients of advanced age: a conservative approach. Laryngoscope 2008;118:270–4.
10. Jackson C, Kaylie D, Coppit G, et al. Glomus jugulare tumors with intracranial extension. Neurosurg Focus 2004;17(2):E7.
11. Woods C, Strasnick B, Jackson C. Surgery for glomus tumors: the otology group experience. Laryngoscope 1993;103(11 Suppl 60):65–72.
12. Jackson C. Diagnosis for treatment planning and treatment options. Laryngoscope 1993;103(Suppl 60):17–22.
13. Erickson D, Kudva Y, Ebersold M, et al. Benign paragangliomas: clinical presentation and treatment outcomes in 236 patients. J Clin Endocrinol Metab 2001;86(11):5210–6.
14. Eldevik O, Gabrielsen T, Jacobsen E. Imaging findings in schwannomas of the jugular foramen. AJNR Am J Neuroradiol 2000;21:1139–44.
15. Olsen W, Dillon W, Kelly W. MR imaging of paragangliomas. Am J Roentgenol 1987;148:201–4.
16. Fisch U. Infratemporal fossa approach for extensive tumors of the temporal bone and base of the skull. In: Silverstein H, Norrel H, editors. Neurological surgery of the ear, vol. 2. Birmingham (England): Aesculapius; 1977. p. 34–53.
17. Glasscock ME III, Jackson C, Harris P. Glomus tumors: diagnosis, classification, and management of large lesions. Arch Otolaryngol 1982;108:409–15.
18. Oldring D, Fisch U. Glomus tumors of the temporal region. Arch Otolaryngol 1981;107:209.
19. Boedeker CC, Neumann H, Offergeld C, et al. Clinical features of paraganglioma syndromes. Skull Base 2009;19(1):17–25.

20. Gaynor BG, Elhammady MS, Jethanamest D, et al. Incidence of cranial nerve palsy after preoperative embolization of glomus jugulare tumors using Onyx. J Neurosurg 2014;120(2):377–81.
21. Sanna M, Jain Y, De Donato G, et al. Management of jugular paragangliomas: the gruppo otologico experience. Otol Neurotol 2004;25:797–804.
22. Bacciu A, Medina M, Ait Mimoune H, et al. Lower cranial nerves function after surgical treatment of Fisch Class C and D tympanojugular paragangliomas. Eur Arch Otorhinolaryngol 2015 Feb;272(2):311–9.
23. Moe KS, Li D, Linder TE, et al. An update on the surgical treatment of temporal bone paraganglioma. Skull Base 1999;9:185–94.
24. Willen SN, Einstein DB, Maciunas RJ, et al. Treatment of glomus jugulare tumors in patients with advanced age: planned limited surgical resection followed by staged gamma knife radiosurgery: a preliminary report. Otol Neurotol 2005;26: 1229–34.
25. Cole JM, Beiler D. Long term results of treatment for glomus jugulare and glomus vagale tumors with radiotherapy. Laryngoscope 1994;104:1461–5.
26. Larner JM, Hahn SS, Spaulding CA, et al. Glomus Jugulare tumors. Long-term control by radiation therapy. Cancer 1992;69:1813–7.
27. Carasco V, Rosenman J. Radiation therapy of glomus jugulare tumors. Laryngoscope 1993;103:23–7.
28. Sheehan JP, Tanaka S, Link M, et al. Gamma Knife surgery for the management of glomus tumors: a multicenter study. J Neurosurg 2012;117:246–54.
29. Ivan ME, Sughrue ME, Clark AJ, et al. A meta-analysis of tumor control creates and treatment-related morbitiy for patients with glomus jugulare tumors. J Neurosurg 2011;114:1299–305.
30. Chen PG, Nyugen JH, Payne SC, et al. Treatment of glomus jugulare tumors with Gamma Knife radiosurgery. Laryngoscope 2010;120:1856–62.
31. Van der Mey AG, Frijns JH, Cornelisse CT, et al. Does intervention improve the natural course of glomus tumors? A series of 108 patietns seen in a 32-year period. Ann Otol Rhinol Laryngol 1992;101(8):635–42.
32. Prasad SC, Mimoune HA, D'Orazio F, et al. The role of wait-and-scan and the efficacy of radiotherapy in the treatment of temporal bone paragangliomas. Otol Neurotol 2014;35(5):922–31.
33. Jackson CG, Haynes DS, Walker PA, et al. Hearing conservation in surgery for glomus jugulare tumors. Am J Otol 1996;17(3):425–37.
34. Wanna GB, Sweeney AD, Carlson ML, et al. Subtotal resection for management of large jugular paragangliomas with functional lower cranial nerves. Otolaryngol Head Neck Surg 2014;151(6):991–5.
35. Carlson ML, Sweeney AD, Wanna GB, et al. Natural history of glomus jugulare: a review of 16 tumors managed with primary observation. Otolaryngol Head Neck Surg 2015;152:98–105.

Nonparaganglioma Jugular Foramen Tumors

Andrew J. Thomas, MD, Richard H. Wiggins III, MD, Richard K. Gurgel, MD*

KEYWORDS

- Jugular foramen • Nonparaganglioma • Jugular foramen schwannoma
- Jugular foramen meningioma • Jugular foramen endolymphatic sac tumor
- Jugular foramen chordoma • Jugular foramen chondrosarcoma

KEY POINTS

- Nonparaganglioma jugular foramen tumors are rare tumors and include schwannomas, meningiomas, endolymphatic sac tumors, chordomas, and chondrosarcomas, and metastatic disease spread to the jugular foramen.
- The clinical presentation of any jugular foramen tumor may include symptoms related to neuropathies of the facial, vestibulocochlear, or lower cranial nerves; pulsatile tinnitus; or audiovestibular symptoms.
- Imaging is crucial in the evaluation of jugular foramen tumors and computed tomography (CT), MRI, and angiography provide complementary information in the diagnosis and preoperative planning for jugular foramen tumors.
- Surgical resection is often the primary treatment of nonparaganglioma jugular foramen tumors; however, the role of adjuvant radiotherapy and primary stereotactic radiotherapy is developing and promising.
- Stereotactic radiotherapy is an important adjuvant when subtotal resection is necessary or in cases of tumor recurrence.

EPIDEMIOLOGY

Jugular paragangliomas are the most common tumors of the jugular foramen (JF) with an incidence of 1 per 1.3 million people per year (250 cases in the United States per year).[1,2] Paragangliomas are not, however, the only tumors found in the JF. Schwannomas, meningiomas, and other tumors also grow in this location, although each is rare. As of 2005, there were only an estimated 200 cases of JF schwannoma reported in the English literature, and less than 100 cases of JF meningioma reported as of 2007.[3,4] Even less common tumors that may involve or extend into the JF include

Disclosures: None.
Division of Otolaryngology, University of Utah, 50 North Medical Drive, Salt Lake City, UT 84132, USA
* Corresponding author.
E-mail address: Richard.Gurgel@hsc.utah.edu

Otolaryngol Clin N Am 48 (2015) 343–359
http://dx.doi.org/10.1016/j.otc.2014.12.008
oto.theclinics.com

Abbreviations	
CN	Cranial nerve
CPA	Cerebellopontine angle
CT	Computed tomography
ELST	Endolymphatic sac tumor
HL	Hearing loss
JF	Jugular foramen
VHL	von Hippel-Lindau

endolymphatic sac tumors (ELST), chordomas, and chondrocytomas, and metastatic disease spread to the JF.

JF schwannomas are rare, with a reported incidence of 2.9% to 4% of all intracranial schwannomas and less than 1% of all temporal bone lesions.[3,5] There are a limited number of small case series and reviews in the literature because of the rarity of these tumors. These tumors are reported to have an increased incidence in women and have an average age of incidence of 37 years.[6] These tumors rarely present before the second or after the seventh decades of life.[6] Presentation in the first or second decade of life should raise clinical suspicion for neurofibromatosis type 2.[5]

JF meningiomas are very rare tumors that represent approximately 0.7% to 4% of all posterior fossa meningiomas. They are the third most common JF tumor following paraganglioma and schwannoma.[4] Meningiomas can originate in the JF or may secondarily involve the JF with expansive growth, such as with some large petroclival meningiomas. Posterior fossa meningiomas are a rare group of tumors themselves, representing approximately 9% to 10% of all intracranial meningiomas. In a series of 161 posterior fossa meningiomas, only seven cases were identified as JF meningiomas.[7] There is a strong female predominance and they usually occur in the fourth or fifth decade of life.[6]

ELSTs are rare, low-grade adenocarcinomas of the endolymphatic sac that may extend through the temporal bone to the JF because of their infiltrative growth pattern.[8] Although most ELSTs occur sporadically, they are a characteristic tumor of von Hippel-Lindau (VHL) disease with an incidence in VHL disease of 11% to 16%.[8–10] VHL disease is an autosomal-dominant tumor syndrome with an incidence of approximately 1 in 36,000 births. The usual age at onset on VHL-associated ELST is in the third decade of life. ELSTs associated with VHL are bilateral in approximately 30% of cases. Sporadic ELST is usually diagnosed at a later age than VHL-associated tumors, and is usually unilateral.[9]

Chordomas and chondrosarcomas are distinct entities but often grouped together because of their similar presentations, radiographic appearance, and anatomic location.[11] These are slow growing, but locally aggressive, and rarely metastasize. Chondrosarcomas are cartilaginous tumors that make up approximately 11% of all bone tumors.[12] Although these tumors are most commonly found in long bones, they involve the head and neck in approximately 10% of cases.[13] They have been reported in a wide range of ages but tend to favor younger patients with no significant gender predilection. When chondrosarcomas involve the skull base they are most likely to arise at the petroclival junction and rarely involve the JF.[12,14] According to a 2008 review by Sanna and colleagues,[14] only 11 cases of chondrosarcoma arising from the JF were reported in the worldwide literature.

Cerebral metastasis occurs in approximately 15% to 35% of patients with cancer.[15,16] In a series of 212 patients with primary nondisseminated malignant neoplasms, 22.2% of the patients were identified to have histopathologic evidence of temporal bone metastasis.[17] Involvement of the skull base has been estimated to occur in approximately 4% of cases of systemic malignancy.[18] Adenocarcinomas that are metastatic to the JF usually originate from the prostate, breast, kidney, or lung.[19]

PRESENTATION

All JF lesions have similar presenting signs and symptoms, which may include neuropathies of the cranial nerves (CNs) V-XII, especially the lower CNs IX-XI and audiovestibular dysfunction.[1] A retrotympanic mass may be seen on otoscopy. Although glomus jugulare tumors are the most common type of JF tumor to present with this constellation of signs and symptoms, JF schwannomas and meningiomas often present similarly.[6]

There are several different JF syndromes that are described based on differential involvement of the lower CNs. Although these syndromes are described as JF syndromes, lesions that cause these symptoms may occur anywhere along the course of the involved nerves from the brainstem to the extracranial site of innervation, not exclusively during their course through the JF. The constellation of lower CN deficits seen in JF syndromes have also been described for etiologies other than JF tumors including brainstem cerebral vascular accident and leptomeningeal processes (including tuberculosis, syphilis, and neurosarcoidosis). Abscess, trauma, and aneurysm may also result in a similar pattern of lower CN deficits.[6]

- JF (Vernet) syndrome: Unilateral involvement of CN IX-XI resulting in loss of taste from the posterior one-third of the tongue; ipsilateral anesthesia of the palate, pharynx, and larynx; and ipsilateral weakness of vocal cords, palate, trapezius, and sternocleidomastoid.
- Posterior lacerocondylar (Collet-Sicard) syndrome: Involvement of IX-XI as in JF syndrome with addition of hypoglossal nerve (CN XII) involvement causing tongue weakness.
- Posterior retropharyngeal (Villaret) syndrome: Involvement of IX-XII as in posterior lacerocondylar syndrome but with the addition of sympathetic chain involvement leading to Horner syndrome.

JF meningiomas often present with hearing loss (HL), tinnitus, and a middle ear mass. Lower CN dysfunction is often present, although single nerve involvement seems to be more common than multiple nerve/JF syndromes.[6] Other presenting signs and symptoms may include a mass in the neck or hoarseness. The presence of conductive HL is often caused by tumor extending into the middle ear and surrounding the ossicles without destruction or erosion, which is characteristic of tegmen tympani and JF meningiomas.[20]

The presentation of JF schwannomas is variable depending on where the bulk of the tumor is located. The tumor may be predominantly intracranial, extracranial, or dumbbell-shaped in both compartments. The most common presentations involve HL, which is reported in up to 60% to 75% of patients, and lower CN deficits, reported in more than 50% of cases. However, if most of the tumor is intracranial with only mild involvement of the JF, the patient may present with minimal or no lower CN deficit and have primarily symptoms associated with intracranial mass including HL, tinnitus, and vertigo.[6] A middle ear mass is rarely seen with these tumors.[3] These tumors can also cause displacement of the facial nerve similar to vestibular schwannomas, and postoperative facial weakness has been reported in 20% to 25% of patients in some series.[6]

The presentation of ELST is nonspecific and may be mistaken for other conditions. Chordomas and chondrosarcomas may present with headaches and diplopia, and trigeminal (CN V) neuropathy may also be present. Lower CN dysfunction is less common than with JF schwannomas and meningiomas.[6]

Metastatic disease behaves more aggressively than JF tumors of benign histology and is more likely to cause cranial neuropathy. Metastatic disease is the most common cause of the JF syndrome.[18] There is usually a rapid onset of symptoms as compared with the more insidious development of symptoms seen with JF paragangliomas, schwannomas, or meningiomas.[21]

EVALUATION AND DIAGNOSIS

Although all JF lesions may have similarities in their clinical presentation, it is important to accurately diagnose the type of lesion. The behavior of the different tumor types is different and there are differences in preoperative evaluation, expected outcomes, and risk of recurrence.[1] Imaging is the cornerstone of the diagnostic process.

Preoperative imaging should include computed tomography (CT) and MRI, which provide complementary data for evaluating lesions of the JF.[3,22] CT is particularly useful for evaluation of the osseous margins and identification of important bony landmarks for surgical planning (**Fig. 1**). CT imaging should be performed with axial thin sections of 1.0 mm or thinner, without contrast, in bone algorithm (maximum edge enhancement), and include coronal reconstruction.[1]

MRI allows for a more detailed evaluation of the tumor and the brain, posterior fossa, and soft tissues of the neck. MRI provides important information about the extension of the JF mass and the potential for evaluating vascular involvement.[1] Evaluation of the skull base with MRI should be performed with axial and coronal thin section (4 mm or thinner) with T1- and T2-weighted sequences, thin section gadolinium-enhanced T1-weighted sequences with fat saturation, and diffusion-weighted sequences. The apparent diffusion coefficient series included with diffusion (diffusion weighted imaging [DWI] or diffusion tensor imaging [DTI]) imaging can be very helpful as a marker of tumor cellularity. Fat saturation is a useful technique for evaluating bone marrow involvement, particularly for tumors that extend into the petrous apex and erode the clivus. Postcontrast thin sections are helpful for tumor spread patterns, such as with perineural invasion, and foramen involvement.[1]

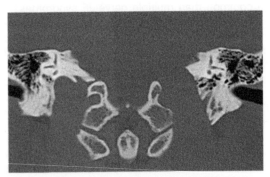

Fig. 1. Coronal CT reconstruction showing a normal right jugular foramen and an abnormal left jugular foramen with smooth scalloped margins, with an almost surgical appearance, consistent with jugular foramen osseous changes from a schwannoma. (*Courtesy of* Amirsys, Inc, Salt Lake City, UT; with permission.)

For vascular lesions of the JF, such as paragangliomas and ELSTs, angiography is also useful.[22] Angiography allows for assessment of the vascularity of the tumor and its relationship to the carotid artery. In the case of carotid artery encasement or occlusion, a balloon test can then be used to predict how well the patient would tolerate ligation of the carotid if necessary. The venous phase of angiography should also be evaluated to determine if there is intraluminal extension of the tumor mass or occlusion of the jugular bulb, jugular vein, or the sigmoid sinus.[22] Moreover, venous angiography can be used to embolize the inferior petrosal sinus, which can minimize blood loss during resection because this sinus is otherwise difficult to manage until the jugular bulb has been opened.[23]

IMAGING CHARACTERISTICS

Meningiomas are solid, well-circumscribed, extra-axial masses. These tumors are usually sessile with a broad dural base because the intracranial spread along the dura is "en plaque" rather than globular in most cases.[24,25] On CT imaging, there is commonly an increase in the density (sclerotic changes) of the bone adjacent to the meningioma (**Fig. 2**). On MRI, there is usually intense, uniform enhancement, with an enhancing dural tail along the margin, and in comparison with glomus jugulare, an absence of flow voids (**Fig. 3**).[1,20] Meningiomas may arise within the JF, or they may originate in the posterior fossa and extend into the JF, termed primary or secondary JF meningiomas, respectively, based on their site of origin.[24,26] Primary JF meningiomas have a unique growth pattern. They tend to be more infiltrative and often

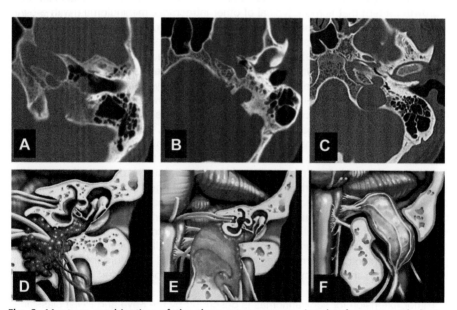

Fig. 2. Montage combination of the three most common jugular foramen pathologies demonstrating the importance of osseous changes found on CT in differentiating these complex pathologies. The first axial CT image (A) shows the permeative changes characteristic of a jugular foramen paraganglioma (D). The middle case (B) shows the increase in bone density that is seen with sclerotic osseous changes found adjacent to a jugular foramen meningioma (E). The final case (C) shows the smooth scalloped surgical margins found with a benign nerve sheath slow-growing lesion enlarging the jugular foramen that is found with a jugular foramen schwannoma (F). (*Courtesy of* Amirsys, Inc, Salt Lake City, UT; with permission.)

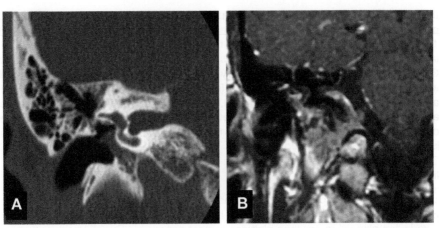

Fig. 3. (*A*) Coronal CT reconstruction through the right middle ear demonstrates soft tissue overlying the cochlear promontory, without osseous destruction. (*B*) Correlating coronal postcontrasted fat-saturated T1 image shows an avidly enhancing extra-axial lesion with dural tails centered at the jugular foramen, consistent with a jugular foramen meningioma. (*Courtesy of* Amirsys, Inc, Salt Lake City, UT; with permission.)

demonstrate a centrifugal growth pattern with expansion of the bony margins of the foramen along with local intraosseous extension.[1] Secondary JF meningiomas have a growth pattern that is more typical of other intracranial meningiomas, with growth characterized by the soft tissue mass component with minimal bone involvement.[24]

Schwannomas typically show a smooth-corticated margin. Schwannomas cause expansion of the JF but do not invade the marrow space.[24] This type of JF expansion is well-visualized on CT. On MRI, schwannomas typically show isointensity on T1, hyperintensity on T2 sequences, and there are no flow voids (distinguishing from glomus jugulare) or dural tails (distinguishing from meningioma). Occasionally, cystic degeneration (intratumoral cysts) may be seen within the schwannoma. Schwannomas avidly enhance on MRI T1 gadolinium-enhanced images.[24] JF schwannomas are typically lobulated, well circumscribed, and elongated following the course of the CNs **(Fig. 2)**.[6] These tumors follow the course of CNs IX-XI, as they arise from these nerves, and therefore extend along the nerves superomedially into the posterior fossa toward the lateral brainstem, or inferiorly toward the nasopharyngeal carotid space. Up to 90% of these tumors are reported to arise from the glossopharyngeal or vagus nerve.[27] A case series of 10 JF schwannomas revealed involvement of these locations with no involvement of the temporal bone or clivus.[24] This constrained spread along the CNs distinguishes JF schwannomas from the infiltration of JF meningiomas and glomus jugulare tumors into the surrounding skull base. Minimal or no tumor blush is seen in these tumors on angiography, which would not typically be indicated if a schwannoma is suspected.

Tumor extension for schwannomas is described by the Kaye and Pellet classification.[28,29] Kaye and colleagues[28] described three classes of JF schwannoma: (1) intracranial with minimal extension into bone (type A), (2) primarily within bone regardless of intracranial component (type B), and (3) primarily extracranial with minimal extension into bone or into the posterior fossa (type C). Pellet and colleagues[29] proposed the addition of a fourth class of JF schwannoma describing dumbbell-shaped tumors with extracranial and intracranial extensions linked via the JF (type D). The type and extent of tumor extension is important to identify on preoperative imaging to identify the optimal surgical approach to the JF that maximizes tumor resection and neural preservation.

Characteristic findings of chordomas or chondrosarcomas that extend to the JF include irregular bony erosion and occasional calcifications within the mass seen on CT, and hypointense or isointense in signal on T1-weighted and hyperintense on T2-weighted MRI. Gadolinium enhancement may be heterogeneous or homogeneous and the tumor may have a "soap bubble" appearance.[30] These pathologies cause expansile changes to the skull base, whereas approximately 50% of chondrosarcomas demonstrate a chondroid matrix within the lesion. Chordomas and chondrosarcomas have a similar radiographic appearance, but the location may distinguish these tumors. Chordomas of the skull base arise in the midline in the clivus, because they originate from notochord remnants. Chondrosarcomas have a more laterally located center and grow toward the midline because they arise from mesenchymal cells or rests of cartilage within the skull base.[11] The value in distinguishing these tumor types relates to differences in prognosis and the role of adjunct radiotherapy.

ELSTs are often confused for other JF lesions based solely on their imaging characteristics that are similar to other infiltrative tumors, such as paragangliomas. These tumors are centered in the endolymphatic sac at the posterior petrous surface, however, and demonstrate a destructive pattern of growth best seen on CT, with central calcification, and a posterior rim of calcification. MRI characteristics of ELSTs typically include hyperintensity on T1-weighted images and heterogeneous enhancement with gadolinium, similar to glomus jugulare, with a "salt and pepper" appearance (**Fig. 4**) from hypervascularity. There is heterogenous hyperintensity on T2-weighted images (see **Fig. 5**).[9]

Characteristic imaging findings for metastatic tumors involving the JF include permeative destruction of the skull base, best seen on CT. This is distinct from the predictable growth of paragangliomas, which spread along a pathway of least resistance. Vascular metastases from primary sites, such as renal and thyroid carcinoma, may

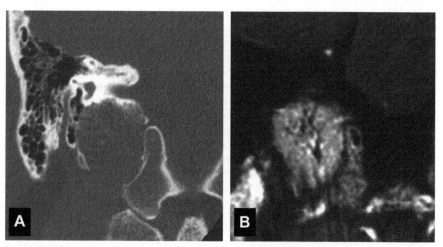

Fig. 4. (A) Coronal CT demonstrates permeative changes surrounding the jugular foramen superiorly and laterally to the jugular foramen. (B) Correlating coronal T1 postcontrasted fat-saturated image shows avid enhancement of the lesion itself, with internal dark linear foci, consistent with the flow voids of the vascularity contained within this paraganglioma, often described as the pepper of these "salt and pepper" lesions. (*Courtesy of* Amirsys, Inc, Salt Lake City, UT; with permission.)

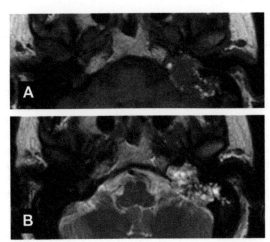

Fig. 5. (A) Axial T1 precontrast image through the jugular foramen shows the bright T1 signal intensity (T1 shortening) within a lesion centered along the left posterior petrous ridge. (B) The correlating axial T2-weighted image shows the expansile nature and T2 bright signal intensity and the multiseptated appearance found with endolymphatic sac tumors. (*Courtesy of* Amirsys, Inc, Salt Lake City, UT; with permission.)

appear similar to paragangliomas, but are differentiated by the particularly destructive growth pattern (**Fig. 6**).[21]

TREATMENT

There are three main management strategies for benign JF lesions: (1) observation, (2) stereotactic radiation, and (3) microsurgical resection. The JF is at the junction of the base of the temporal bone and the occipital bone inferior to the otic capsule.[31,32] Although it is termed the jugular "foramen" the anatomic structure is actually a canal. Following the canal out of the skull base, it courses anterior, lateral, and then inferior.[33] The JF is one of the most variable structures of the skull base. Anatomic relationships to the jugular bulb include a fibrous sheath investing the jugular bulb and intimately related with the carotid sheath, the intrapetrous course of the internal carotid artery (segment C2) positioned anterior to the JF, the otic capsule superior to the JF, the facial nerve descending segment posterior and lateral to the JF, and the posterior fossa medial and posterior to the JF. Laterally the jugular bulb is also divided from the facial nerve by retrofacial and infralabyrinthine air cells.[32]

The anteromedial portion of the JF has been described by Rhoton and Buza[34] as the pars nervosa, which contains CN IX and the inferior petrosal sinus. The posterolateral portion has been described as the pars venosa containing CN X and XI and the jugular bulb.[31,34,35] The foramen often exists as a single compartment; however, there is occasionally a fibrous, and less commonly an osseous septum dividing it into posterolateral and anteromedial compartments.[31,34,36] The tympanic branch of CN IX (Jacobson nerve) and the auricular branch of CN X (Arnold nerve) emerge from within the JF.

Microsurgery

Choosing an appropriate surgical approach to the JF depends on the type and extent of the tumor. The best approach is one that provides maximum exposure with minimal morbidity and allows for control of neurovascular structures and resection of the tumor in its entirety.[22] The approaches can be categorized by their anatomic relationship to

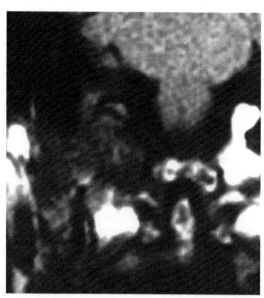

Fig. 6. Coronal noncontrasted T1-weighted MRI without fat saturation shows the normal bright T1 signal intensity within the osseous structures surrounding the left jugular foramen, such as the occipital condyle, whereas the jugular foramen metastatic focus surrounding the right jugular foramen demonstrates dark signal intensity consistent with a marrow-replacing process. (*Courtesy of* Amirsys, Inc, Salt Lake City, UT; with permission.)

the JF, either lateral, posterior, or anterior. Lateral approaches include the infratemporal fossa approach (Fisch type A) and transmastoid transjugular approaches. The posterior approaches include the posterior fossa approaches, such as the retrosigmoid and suboccipital approaches, far lateral, and transcondylar approaches. The anterior approaches include the subtemporal-middle fossa and the infratemporal fossa approaches (Fisch type B and C). Important considerations in selecting the appropriate approach for a given JF lesion include the specific type of tumor, the origin of the tumor, and its degree of extension; the relationship of the tumor to surrounding vasculature, vascular supply to the tumor, and the patency or involvement of surrounding venous outflow; neurologic involvement of the lower CNs, brainstem compression, and any associated hydrocephalus.[22]

Tumors that are primarily intracranial with intact hearing (type A schwannomas and cerebellopontine angle [CPA] meningiomas) may be accessed with a posterior approach, such as a retrosigmoid craniotomy with preservation of the external and internal auditory canals.[3,7,22] For a large posterior fossa component a translabyrinthine approach may be necessary, and depending on the extent of extension into the JF may be combined with an infratemporal fossa approach.[3] Depending on the caudal extent of the intracranial portion of the tumor, a far lateral or extreme lateral approach may be indicated for better access to the foramen magnum.[7] For tumors that have significant extension into the JF (type B schwannomas) a lateral transjugular approach (with or without craniotomy) or the Fisch type A infratemporal fossa approach with facial nerve rerouting in particular, provides the best exposure of the JF extent of the tumor.[22] An alternative to routing the facial nerve, known as the "fallopian bridge" technique, is also reasonable to use and minimizes trauma from manipulation of the facial nerve.[37] The infratemporal fossa approach provides exposure of the JF, carotid artery, and the temporal bone in addition to allowing access into the posterior fossa.[3] For primarily extracranial tumors (type C schwannomas) the location of the tumor dictates the most appropriate approach; transcondylar or far lateral approaches may provide better exposure for tumors inferior to the jugular bulb, and infratemporal fossa approaches are preferable for tumors lateral and anterior to the bulb. For tumors with significant intracranial and extracranial components (dumbbell-shaped or type D schwannomas) infratemporal and posterior fossa exposure can be obtained with a combination of the infratemporal fossa approach (Fisch type A) and a retrosigmoid approach.[3,22]

Infratemporal fossa approach (Fisch type A)

There are multiple variants of the infratemporal fossa approach developed by Fisch, which are termed Fisch A, B, and C. The original reports by Fisch are filled with excellent descriptions and illustrations of these procedures.[38] The type A approach provides access to the infralabyrinthine and petrous apex/pyramid tip, the type B approach to the clivus, and the type C approach to the parasellar and parasphenoid regions. The type A approach, with modification to the originally described facial nerve transposition technique, is the most commonly used. The infratemporal fossa approach is ideal for large JF lesions because it provides superior exposure to other techniques that do not remove the external auditory canal or reroute the facial nerve. It may also be modified and combined with other approaches depending on the extent and specific involvement of the tumor. It provides exposure of the JF and the infralabyrinthine region, and is used for tumors invading the infralabyrinthine and apical temporal bone or with intradural extension. The basic steps of the infratemporal fossa exposure are managing the external auditory canal with removal of the tympanic portion of the temporal bone, performing a complete mastoidectomy, transposing the facial nerve, performing a neck dissection with isolation of the lower CNs and great vessels, resecting the tumor, and closing the wound.[32]

The fallopian bridge technique is a modification of the infratemporal fossa approach, which omits taking down the canal wall and leaves the facial nerve skeletonized within the fallopian bridge. This technique can decrease the risk of postoperative facial nerve dysfunction and conductive HL. This technique provides adequate exposure for tumor resection in most cases.[37,39,40] The fallopian bridge technique may be particularly well suited to JF schwannoma resection because these tumors originate medially in the jugular bulb and expand without infiltrating vasculature.[39]

Translabyrinthine approach

The translabyrinthine approach is particularly useful for JF tumors with a large posterior fossa component and nonservicable hearing. The obvious downside to this procedure is the sacrifice of any residual hearing, which makes patient selection important in regard to preoperative hearing and anticipated postoperative hearing. Advantages of this approach include excellent exposure of the facial nerve and wide exposure of the CPA.[41]

Transcochlear approach

The transcochlear approach provides access to the CPA with the most direct exposure of the prepontine cisterns and the midclivus. This technique may be useful for JF tumors with a large CPA component in the prepontine area. This is particularly useful for meningiomas extending from the midline where the transcochlear approach offers unique ability to access and control the base of implantation and blood supply. The advantages of the transcochlear approach must be weighed against resulting morbidity from complete unilateral HL, vestibulopathy, and temporary facial weakness from facial nerve rerouting. This approach is appropriate when there is already no service for complete tumor removal. The transotic approach is an alternative to the transcochlear approach, distinguished by leaving the facial nerve in a fallopian bridge, rather than being rerouted.

Retrosigmoid craniotomy

The retrosigmoid craniotomy allows for hearing preservation as opposed to the transcochlear or translabyrinthine approaches to the CPA. This approach is particularly relevant for nonparaganglioma JF tumors that are primarily located in the inferior CPA with minimal extension into the JF, and particularly in cases of intact hearing on the operative side. This approach offers the best exposure of the inferior CPA including the JF to the foramen magnum, but provides inadequate lateral exposure for approaching tumors with significant temporal bone invasion.[42]

Ideally, JF tumors should be removed completely and neurovascular structures preserved. However, this is not always possible because of unacceptable complications from resection of CNs, involvement of critical vascular structures, patient age, or inability to undergo surgery. If subtotal resection or avoidance of surgery is necessary, stereotactic radiosurgery may be an option particularly for schwannomas.[43,44] Complete resection of meningiomas should be attempted whenever possible because they have a particularly high rate of recurrence, likely because of their bony invasion of the skull base.[26] Schwannomas have a decreased likelihood of recurrence compared with meningioma, and therefore a more conservative approach can be taken. In a series of 81 patients with JF schwannomas, a conservative approach to resection (72.1% near-total resections in the conservative approach group and 9.4% near-total resections in the standard treatment group) led to a significant decrease in CN deficits with no significant increase in recurrence.[44]

Complete resection of ELST is advisable over subtotal resection because of their malignant nature. Additionally, recurrence after a subtotal resection is more likely to result in larger multifocal disease compared with a more easily managed focal recurrence after a gross total resection.[8] Chordoma and chondrosarcoma are both slow-growing tumors that rarely metastasize, and the primary goal of treatment is to establish complete surgical resection.[14] Patients with a single metastatic brain lesion to the JF are most likely to benefit from surgery if the lesion can be completely resected, they have minimal or no evident extracranial disease, and demonstrate good performance status.[15] Postoperative radiation is typically recommended after resection.

Potential surgical complications include cerebrospinal fluid leak, wound infection, and meningitis. The incidence of cerebrospinal fluid leak is consistent with rates for other skull base approaches, with a reported range of 3.9% to 6.6%.[45] A lumbar drain may be used to manage postoperative cerebrospinal fluid leak. The risk of cerebrospinal fluid leak can be reduced by first ensuring appropriate dural closure, using a free fat graft to fill the extradural defect, or using a regional or free muscle flap if needed.[28,45] Other potential postoperative complications include neurologic deficits related to CNs VII-XII or the sympathetic chain. The most common early complication seen is vocal cord paralysis, which in this same series occurred in 25% to 33% of the patients, with late complications related to dysfunction of the lower CNs including speech and swallowing dysfunction and shoulder dysfunction or pain.[45] The mortality rate may be as low as 1%, with most major series reporting no mortalities related to JF tumor resection.[46]

Radiotherapy

Stereotactic radiotherapy has been promising in vestibular schwannoma and has recently been applied to nonvestibular schwannomas.[43,44] Recent studies of radiation for vestibular schwannoma have demonstrated excellent tumor control with decreased CN morbidity, although robust long-term outcome data are still needed.[47] For radiation performed in the absence of microsurgery, it has been reported that 47% of patients had improvement in lower CN function at a median of 16 months postradiation, and 21% of all patients including those who had previous microsurgery.[46] Stereotactic radiation has been specifically recommended for small or medium sized JF schwannomas without any brainstem mass effect and in older patients or those who cannot undergo surgery. Based on limited long-term follow-up data for patients with JF schwannomas treated with stereotactic radiation, results have been promising with low morbidity, adequate tumor control, CN preservation, and in some cases reversal of cranial neuropathies.[44,48]

Stereotactic radiation can also be effectively used to treat JF meningiomas for patients in whom surgery or observation are not the best options. Radiotherapy may also be used as an adjunct to surgery for unresectable residual disease.[1] Recent studies on the use of stereotactic radiation for skull base and posterior fossa meningiomas have shown promising results. Local control rates of 92% to 100% have been reported after stereotactic radiation for skull base meningiomas, with doses that would be appropriate for JF lesions. The incidence of permanent deficits in these studies was 1.6% to 9.8%.[49] In a study of 255 patients receiving radiation for meningiomas of the skull base, progression-free survival of 96% and 78% at 5 and 10 years was achieved. Only 8.6% of patients in this study developed new-onset cranial neuropathies.[50] There is a theoretic advantage to use of proton therapy for larger tumors and those more intimately associated with important neurologic structures. However, overall toxicity and tumor control with proton therapy for meningiomas has been similar to photon therapy.[51] For tumors with subtotal resection, stereotactic radiation should only be used when there is documented growth of the residual tumor on serial imaging. This strategy minimizes unnecessary use of radiation therapy for nongrowing tumor remnants and potential risk for radiation-related morbidity.

There are limited data on the effectiveness of primary radiation therapy for ELST and no added benefit has been demonstrated for postoperative adjuvant radiotherapy in regard to control of residual tumor growth and recurrence rates.[52,53] In cases of incomplete resection, radiation therapy may add some benefit but available data on outcomes are mixed and the results are inconclusive.[8,53] Stereotactic proton and photon radiotherapy have been used as adjuvant treatment of chordoma and chondrosarcoma. Primary radiotherapy is not recommended for these tumors (unless contraindications exist to surgery) because surgical resection after radiation would be particularly challenging and improved results are seen with radiation therapy following maximal tumor resection. For chondrosarcomas of the JF, Sanna and colleagues[14] recommended reserving postoperative adjuvant radiation therapy for recurrent tumor after surgical resection, subtotal resection, or for tumors more aggressive than grade I. For metastatic disease to the JF, whole-brain radiation therapy is often recommended with or without surgical excision. The standard dose fractionation is 3000 cGy in 10 fractions daily.[54] For patients unable to undergo surgical excision and standard radiotherapy, stereotactic radiation to the metastasis may provide benefit in neurologic palliation and potentially long-term tumor control of a metastatic lesion but these data are limited.[55,56]

Observation

Observation of JF schwannomas or meningiomas is a reasonable option for older patients, those with small tumors, or for patients who have medical contraindications to surgery. If these benign JF tumors show interval growth on serial imaging, intervention by means of surgery or radiation may be warranted. Observation of ELST is not appropriate because these are locally aggressive adenocarcinomas that are best treated with early surgical resection. Delayed resection risks increasing difficulty of gross total resection and morbidity related to neurovascular involvement.[8] For metastatic disease to the JF, observation alone following whole-brain radiation therapy may be indicated for patients who are not surgical candidates. For chordoma and chondrosarcoma watchful waiting has been suggested as a reasonable conservative approach for asymptomatic lesions, with close follow-up imaging to assess growth of the lesion. For rapid growth or development of symptoms surgical resection and radiation can then be planned.[30] For chondrosarcoma, a 10- to 15-year follow-up or longer has been recommended because some cases of recurrence may present much later, even 20 to 30 years after treatment.[13,57]

For all types of JF tumors mentioned, close observation after surgical resection is necessary to monitor for residual progressive disease. Because of the slow-growing nature of schwannomas and meningiomas, long-term follow-up is particularly important to identify recurrence. Follow-up consists of clinical examination and serial MRIs. Extent of the initial tumor resection is also considered in determining length of follow-up. Patients with subtotal resection are followed with clinical and MRI surveillance indefinitely, although the interval between serial scans can be lengthened if there is no evidence of growth on early serial imaging. There is no evidence-based protocol for duration of follow-up, but a reasonable approach with observation could include annual imaging, lengthened to imaging every 2 to 3 years after a period of no growth, eventually lengthened to every 5 years if there is sustained quiescence.

OUTCOMES
Recurrence

JF meningiomas have a tendency to recur. This is thought to be related to bony invasion into the skull base, which may evade resection. Wide exposure and resection of involved bone therefore is appropriate for minimizing chance of recurrence. For JF meningiomas, a 25% overall recurrence rate has been reported at 5-year follow-up.[1,26] However, this rate depends on the grade of resection achieved; for Simpson grade I resection of intracranial meningiomas a 5-year recurrence rate of 4% has been reported. Stereotactic radiation may be given to control growth of residual tumor.

JF schwannomas are less likely to recur than meningiomas. In a surgical series of 81 patients with JF schwannomas, there was an 8.9% (six patients) recurrence rate. There was a nonsignificant trend toward increased recurrence in patients with subtotal resection of JF schwannoma followed by stereotactic radiation but a clear reduction in morbidity, leading the authors of this study to conclude that the risks of recurrence with subtotal resection followed by stereotactic radiation are outweighed by reduced postoperative neuropathies. More data are available on vestibular schwannoma recurrence where the recurrence rate is estimated to be approximately 3% (up to 11%), for both gross total resection and near total resection. However, the rate of recurrence increases to approximately 32% to 53% in cases of subtotal resection depending on the extent of resection.[47,58]

Chondrosarcomas are associated with decreased incidence of recurrence and better long-term control compared with chordomas.[11] The disease-specific survival after surgical resection of skull base chondrosarcoma is approximately 70% at 10 years.[13,57] Chordomas, and the chondroid chordoma variant, are associated with a generally aggressive disease course, a high rate of disease recurrence, and poor outcomes for recurrent disease.[11]

A 90% cure rate has been reported for complete surgical resection of ELSTs.[10] ELST metastasis is extremely rare with only four cases known to be reported in the literature.[59–62] Recurrence has been reported to be more likely with sporadic cases of ELST than with VHL-associated tumors because sporadic cases are more aggressive in nature.[9]

Cranial Neuropathy

The incidence of new postoperative lower CN dysfunction is greatest for JF meningiomas, followed by glomus jugulare tumors, then JF schwannomas occurring in approximately 50% to 60%, 18.9% to 30%, and 15% to 22.2% of cases, respectively.[1,6,45,63,64] This is opposite from the preoperative incidence of lower CN dysfunction, which is greatest for schwannoma, followed by meningioma and glomus jugulare.[63] Transposition of the facial nerve may cause a moderate postoperative paresis, which typically improves in 3 to 12 months.[65] If transposition can be avoided, postoperative facial nerve palsy can be mitigated in most cases.[39] Overall, most patients experience normal or near-normal facial nerve function with more than 88.1% House-Brackmann I or II facial function reported for a series of 83 JF tumors (67 glomus jugulare, 9 schwannomas, 7 meningiomas) with the best long-term facial nerve outcomes seen in glomus jugulare tumors and the poorest in meningiomas.[45] A series of 13 JF meningiomas reported 46.1% House-Brackmann I or II function postoperatively.[4]

Chondrosarcoma of the JF is associated with a high postoperative incidence of CN IX and X deficit, based on a limited number of cases.[14] Metastatic disease in the JF is associated with rapid onset of multiple lower CN dysfunction.[18,21] There are limited data on expected outcomes of CN function after resection but given the invasive nature of metastatic lesions in the JF, preoperative neurologic dysfunction suggests a poor prognosis following resection. For radiation planning, it is recommended that dose delivered to CNs be kept lower than 60 Gy to reduce risk of CN dysfunction.[66]

SUMMARY

Nonparaganglioma JF tumors are rare and most frequently include lower CN schwannomas, meningiomas, ELSTs, chordomas, and chondrosarcomas, and metastatic disease. Among the three most common JF lesions, the preoperative incidence of lower CN dysfunction is greatest for JF schwannomas, followed by meningiomas and glomus jugulare tumors. Imaging plays a crucial role in the diagnosis and preoperative planning for these lesions. Imaging should include CT and contrast-enhanced MRI. For highly vascular lesions, angiography should also be used to evaluate the vascularity of the tumor and its relationship to the carotid artery.

Observation, radiation, and microsurgical resection are all viable management options for benign JF tumors. Treatment choice depends on many factors including tumor size, patient preference, CN status, patient age, and medical comorbidities. Selection of the specific surgical approach for a given JF lesion must take into account many factors including tumor type and extent, and the relationship of the lesion to surrounding vasculature and lower CNs. The incidence of new postoperative lower CN dysfunction is greatest for meningioma, followed by glomus jugulare, then schwannoma. The role of adjuvant stereotactic radiotherapy is evolving with promising results from recent studies.

REFERENCES

1. Gilbert ME, Shelton C, McDonald A, et al. Meningioma of the jugular foramen: glomus jugulare mimic and surgical challenge. Laryngoscope 2004;114(1):25–32.

2. Moffat DA, Hardy DG. Surgical management of large glomus jugulare tumours: infra- and trans-temporal approach. J Laryngol Otol 1989;103(12):1167–80.
3. Wilson MA, Hillman TA, Wiggins RH, et al. Jugular foramen schwannomas: diagnosis, management, and outcomes. Laryngoscope 2005;115(8):1486–92.
4. Sanna M, Bacciu A, Falcioni M, et al. Surgical management of jugular foramen meningiomas: a series of 13 cases and review of the literature. Laryngoscope 2007;117(10):1710–9.
5. Samii M, Babu RP, Tatagiba M, et al. Surgical treatment of jugular foramen schwannomas. J Neurosurg 1995;82(6):924–32.
6. Kryzanski JT, Heilman CB. Clinicopathologic features of jugular foramen tumors. Operat Tech Neurosurg 2005;8(1):6–12.
7. Roberti F, Sekhar LN, Kalavakonda C, et al. Posterior fossa meningiomas: surgical experience in 161 cases. Surg Neurol 2001;56(1):8–20 [discussion: 20–1].
8. Carlson ML, Thom JJ, Driscoll CL, et al. Management of primary and recurrent endolymphatic sac tumors. Otol Neurotol 2013;34(5):939–43.
9. Nevoux J, Nowak C, Vellin JF, et al. Management of endolymphatic sac tumors: sporadic cases and von Hippel-Lindau disease. Otol Neurotol 2014;35(5):899–904.
10. Virk JS, Randhawa PS, Saeed SR. Endolymphatic sac tumour: case report and literature review. J Laryngol Otol 2013;127(4):408–10.
11. Almefty K, Pravdenkova S, Colli BO, et al. Chordoma and chondrosarcoma: similar, but quite different, skull base tumors. Cancer 2007;110(11):2457–67.
12. Harvey SA, Wiet RJ, Kazan R. Chondrosarcoma of the jugular foramen. Am J Otol 1994;15(2):257–63.
13. Hong P, Taylor SM, Trites JR, et al. Chondrosarcoma of the head and neck: report of 11 cases and literature review. J Otolaryngol Head Neck Surg 2009;38(2): 279–85.
14. Sanna M, Bacciu A, Pasanisi E, et al. Chondrosarcomas of the jugular foramen. Laryngoscope 2008;118(10):1719–28.
15. Mintz A, Perry J, Spithoff K, et al. Management of single brain metastasis: a practice guideline. Curr Oncol 2007;14(4):131–43.
16. Paek SH, Audu PB, Sperling MR, et al. Reevaluation of surgery for the treatment of brain metastases: review of 208 patients with single or multiple brain metastases treated at one institution with modern neurosurgical techniques. Neurosurgery 2005;56(5):1021–34 [discussion: 1021–34].
17. Gloria-Cruz TI, Schachern PA, Paparella MM, et al. Metastases to temporal bones from primary nonsystemic malignant neoplasms. Arch Otolaryngol Head Neck Surg 2000;126(2):209–14.
18. Hayward D, Morgan C, Emami B, et al. Jugular foramen syndrome as initial presentation of metastatic lung cancer. J Neurol Surg Rep 2012;73(1):14–8.
19. Balasubramaniam S, Deshpande RB, Misra BK. Gamma knife radiosurgery in jugular foramen endolymphatic sac adenocarcinoma. J Clin Neurosci 2009; 16(5):710–1.
20. Hamilton BE, Salzman KL, Patel N, et al. Imaging and clinical characteristics of temporal bone meningioma. AJNR Am J Neuroradiol 2006;27(10):2204–9.
21. Caldemeyer KS, Mathews VP, Azzarelli B, et al. The jugular foramen: a review of anatomy, masses, and imaging characteristics. Radiographics 1997;17(5):1123–39.
22. David CA. Preoperative planning and surgical approaches to tumors of the jugular foramen. Operat Tech Neurosurg 2005;8(1):19–24.
23. Warren FM III, McCool RR, Hunt JO, et al. Preoperative embolization of the inferior petrosal sinus in surgery for glomus jugulare tumors. Otol Neurotol 2011;32(9): 1538–41.

24. Macdonald AJ, Salzman KL, Harnsberger HR, et al. Primary jugular foramen me-ningioma: imaging appearance and differentiating features. AJR Am J Roent-genol 2004;182(2):373–7.
25. Toyama C, Santiago Gebrim EM, Brito R, et al. Primary jugular foramen meningioma. Otol Neurotol 2008;29(3):417–8.
26. Molony TB, Brackmann DE, Lo WW. Meningiomas of the jugular foramen. Otolar-yngol Head Neck Surg 1992;106(2):128–36.
27. Song MH, Lee HY, Jeon JS, et al. Jugular foramen schwannoma: analysis on its origin and location. Otol Neurotol 2008;29(3):387–91.
28. Kaye AH, Hahn JF, Kinney SE, et al. Jugular foramen schwannomas. J Neurosurg 1984;60(5):1045–53.
29. Pellet W, Cannoni M, Pech A. The widened transcochlear approach to jugular foramen tumors. J Neurosurg 1988;69(6):887–94.
30. Lustig LR, Sciubba J, Holliday MJ. Chondrosarcomas of the skull base and temporal bone. J Laryngol Otol 2007;121(8):725–35.
31. Inserra MM, Pfister M, Jackler RK. Anatomy involved in the jugular foramen approach for jugulotympanic paraganglioma resection. Neurosurg Focus 2004; 17(2):E6.
32. Kveton JF. Anatomy of the jugular foramen: the neurotologic perspective. Operat Tech Otolaryngol Head Neck Surg 1996;7(2):95–8.
33. Tekdemir I, Tuccar E, Aslan A, et al. Comprehensive microsurgical anatomy of the jugular foramen and review of terminology. J Clin Neurosci 2001;8(4):351–6.
34. Rhoton AL Jr, Buza R. Microsurgical anatomy of the jugular foramen. J Neurosurg 1975;42(5):541–50.
35. Van Loveren HR, Sing Liu S, Pensak ML, et al. Anatomy of the jugular foramen: the neurosurgical perspective. Operat Tech Otolaryngol Head Neck Surg 1996; 7(2):90–4.
36. Tekdemir I, Tuccar E, Aslan A, et al. The jugular foramen: a comparative radioa-natomic study. Surg Neurol 1998;50(6):557–62.
37. Pensak ML, Jackler RK. Removal of jugular foramen tumors: the fallopian bridge technique. Otolaryngol Head Neck Surg 1997;117(6):586–91.
38. Fisch U, Pillsbury HC. Infratemporal fossa approach to lesions in the temporal bone and base of the skull. Arch Otolaryngol 1979;105(2):99–107.
39. Cokkeser Y, Brackmann DE, Fayad JN. Conservative facial nerve management in jugular foramen schwannomas. Am J Otol 2000;21(2):270–4.
40. Oghalai JS, Leung MK, Jackler RK, et al. Transjugular craniotomy for the man-agement of jugular foramen tumors with intracranial extension. Otol Neurotol 2004;25(4):570–9 [discussion: 579].
41. Brackmann DE, Shelton C, Arriaga MA. Otologic surgery. 3rd edition. Philadel-phia (PA): Saunders; 2010.
42. Yates PD, Jackler RK, Satar B, et al. Is it worthwhile to attempt hearing preserva-tion in larger acoustic neuromas? Otol Neurotol 2003;24(3):460–4.
43. Cavalcanti DD, Martirosyan NL, Verma K, et al. Surgical management and outcome of schwannomas in the craniocervical region. J Neurosurg 2011;114(5):1257–67.
44. Sedney CL, Nonaka Y, Bulsara KR, et al. Microsurgical management of jugular foramen schwannomas. Neurosurgery 2013;72(1):42–6 [discussion: 46].
45. Fayad JN, Keles B, Brackmann DE. Jugular foramen tumors: clinical characteris-tics and treatment outcomes. Otol Neurotol 2010;31(2):299–305.
46. Martin JJ, Kondziolka D, Flickinger JC, et al. Cranial nerve preservation and out-comes after stereotactic radiosurgery for jugular foramen schwannomas. Neuro-surgery 2007;61(1):76–81 [discussion: 81].

47. van de Langenberg R, Hanssens PE, van Overbeeke JJ, et al. Management of large vestibular schwannoma. Part I. Planned subtotal resection followed by Gamma Knife surgery: radiological and clinical aspects. J Neurosurg 2011;115(5):875–84.

48. Suri A, Bansal S, Singh M, et al. Jugular foramen schwannomas: a single institution patient series. J Clin Neurosci 2014;21(1):73–7.

49. Combs SE, Ganswindt U, Foote RL, et al. State-of-the-art treatment alternatives for base of skull meningiomas: complementing and controversial indications for neurosurgery, stereotactic and robotic based radiosurgery or modern fractionated radiation techniques. Radiat Oncol 2012;7:226.

50. Starke RM, Williams BJ, Hiles C, et al. Gamma knife surgery for skull base meningiomas. J Neurosurg 2012;116(3):588–97.

51. Minniti G, Amichetti M, Enrici RM. Radiotherapy and radiosurgery for benign skull base meningiomas. Radiat Oncol 2009;4:42.

52. Husseini ST, Piccirillo E, Taibah A, et al. The Gruppo Otologico experience of endolymphatic sac tumor. Auris Nasus Larynx 2013;40(1):25–31.

53. Kim HJ, Hagan M, Butman JA, et al. Surgical resection of endolymphatic sac tumors in von Hippel-Lindau disease: findings, results, and indications. Laryngoscope 2013;123(2):477–83.

54. Tsao MN, Lloyd N, Wong RK, et al. Whole brain radiotherapy for the treatment of newly diagnosed multiple brain metastases. Cochrane Database Syst Rev 2012;(4):CD003869.

55. Nieder C, Grosu AL, Gaspar LE. Stereotactic radiosurgery (SRS) for brain metastases: a systematic review. Radiat Oncol 2014;9(1):155.

56. Yomo S, Hayashi M. A minimally invasive treatment option for large metastatic brain tumors: long-term results of two-session Gamma Knife stereotactic radiosurgery. Radiat Oncol 2014;9:132.

57. Koch BB, Karnell LH, Hoffman HT, et al. National cancer database report on chondrosarcoma of the head and neck. Head Neck 2000;22(4):408–25.

58. Milligan BD, Pollock BE, Foote RL, et al. Long-term tumor control and cranial nerve outcomes following gamma knife surgery for larger-volume vestibular schwannomas. J Neurosurg 2012;116(3):598–604.

59. Bambakidis NC, Rodrigue T, Megerian CA, et al. Endolymphatic sac tumor metastatic to the spine. Case report. J Neurosurg Spine 2005;3(1):68–70.

60. Ferreira MA, Feiz-Erfan I, Zabramski JM, et al. Endolymphatic sac tumor: unique features of two cases and review of the literature. Acta Neurochir (Wien) 2002; 144(10):1047–53.

61. Robson AK, Eveson JW, Smith IM, et al. Papillary adenocarcinoma of the middle ear. J Laryngol Otol 1990;104(11):915–6.

62. Tay KY, Yu E, Kassel E. Spinal metastasis from endolymphatic sac tumor. AJNR Am J Neuroradiol 2007;28(4):613–4.

63. Lustig LR, Jackler RK. The variable relationship between the lower cranial nerves and jugular foramen tumors: implications for neural preservation. Am J Otol 1996; 17(4):658–68.

64. Ramina R, Neto MC, Fernandes YB, et al. Meningiomas of the jugular foramen. Neurosurg Rev 2006;29(1):55–60.

65. Coscarella E, Tummala RP, Morcos JJ. Infratemporal Fossa Approaches to the Jugular Foramen. Operat Tech Neurosurg 2005;8(1):25–30.

66. Hauptman JS, Barkhoudarian G, Safaee M, et al. Challenges in linear accelerator radiotherapy for chordomas and chondrosarcomas of the skull base: focus on complications. Int J Radiat Oncol Biol Phys 2012;83(2):542–51.

Cholesterol Granuloma and Other Petrous Apex Lesions

Brandon Isaacson, MD

KEYWORDS

- Cholesterol granuloma • Petrous apex • Temporal bone • Skull base • Petrous bone
- Cholesterin granuloma

KEY POINTS

- Petrous apex cholesterol granuloma has a unique appearance on MRI that distinguishes it from other lesions. These lesions are hyperintense on both T1 and T2 weighted images.
- Asymptomatic petrous apex cholesterol granulomas can be managed with observation using serial imaging.
- A thorough headache history should be obtained to determine if this symptom is a result of the more common entities of migraine or muscle tension as opposed to a petrous apex cholesterol granuloma.
- Symptomatic lesions can be managed with marsupialization, with either an endonasal approach or a lateral transtemporal approach, depending on the individual's anatomy.
- Symptom resolution or improvement is achieved in the vast majority of patients regardless of the surgical approach, and one should consider recurrent symptoms or enlargement of the cholesterol granuloma as opposed to lack of aeration in determining disease progression.

INTRODUCTION

Diagnosis and management of petrous apex lesions present unique challenges secondary to their centralized location and critical adjacent and in situ structures. The petrous apex forms the most medial aspect of the temporal bone and is defined laterally by the otic capsule, petrous carotid artery, and the semicanal of the tensor tympani muscle. The superior surface of the petrous apex is the floor of the middle fossa, and it extends from the arcuate eminence to Meckel cave. The posterior surface of the petrous bone extends from the endolymphatic duct operculum to the clivus. The jugular fossa, vertical petrous carotid canal, and inferior petrosal sinus make up the inferior border of the petrous bone. The superior petrosal sinus defines the border

Disclosures: Medical advisory board member and consultant for Advanced Bionics, course instructor for Stryker, consultant for Medtronic.
Department of Otolaryngology—Head and Neck Surgery, University of Texas Southwestern Medical Center, 5323 Harry Hines Boulevard, Dallas, TX 75390-9035, USA
E-mail address: Brandon.isaacson@utsouthwestern.edu

Otolaryngol Clin N Am 48 (2015) 361–373
http://dx.doi.org/10.1016/j.otc.2014.12.009
oto.theclinics.com
0030-6665/15/$ – see front matter © 2015 Elsevier Inc. All rights reserved.

Abbreviations	
CSF	Cerebrospinal fluid
CT	Computed tomography
MRI	Magnetic resonance imaging

between the middle and posterior fossa surface of the petrous apex. The internal auditory canal arbitrarily divides the petrous apex into anterior and posterior segments when viewed from above, which is important with respect to selecting surgical approaches. Petrous apex cholesterol granuloma is a non-neoplastic inflammatory lesion of the petrous apex that is often found incidentally on cranial imaging.[1,2]

EPIDEMIOLOGY AND PATHOPHYSIOLOGY

Asymmetric pneumatization and effusion are the most common entities identified on medical imaging of the petrous apex. It has been estimated that petrous apex effusions outnumber cholesterol granulomas 500 to 1.[3] The incidence of petrous apex cholesterol granuloma has been estimated at 0.6 cases per 1 million population.[4] Cholesterol granulomas are 10 times more common than petrous apex cholesteatomas.[5]

Two hypotheses exist for the pathogenesis of cholesterol granuloma. Uniform to both hypotheses is that blood enters a mucosalized space, and the anaerobic breakdown products of blood, including cholesterol crystals, incite a foreign body giant cell reaction, thus resulting in cyst formation. The original theory proposes that negative pressure resulting from eustachian tube function is responsible for bleeding into a mucosalized space. Jackler and Cho proposed an alternative hypothesis, as middle ear hemorrhage and a hyperpneumatized temporal bone are rarely seen in patients with chronic eustachian tube dysfunction.[6] Another argument by these same authors against the classic hypothesis is that once the air cell is filled with blood, pressure should be equalized, thus no further bleeding would occur, which is necessary for further expansion and enlargement of a cholesterol granuloma. Jackler and Cho offered an alternative exposed marrow hypothesis that cholesterol granulomas form when there is an osseous dehiscence between bone marrow and a pneumatized air cell. They supported this theory by demonstrating that 6 out of 13 patients with cholesterol granuloma indeed had an osseous dehiscence between bone marrow and an air cell in the contralateral petrous apex, whereas control patients with pneumatized petrous apices had no evidence of dehiscence.[6] The exposed marrow theory has been supported by additional temporal bone histologic studies.[7]

PRESENTATION

Petrous apex pathology can present with a variety of symptoms, but is often incidentally discovered on imaging for unrelated symptoms. Headaches, hearing loss, ear pressure, and dizziness are common chief complaints from otolaryngology patients, and these complaints can also be seen in patients with petrous apex lesions. Most headache and petrous apex pathologies are not related to the lesion but are more commonly secondary muscle tension or migraines. Retro orbital pain and generalized temporoparietal headaches are sometimes seen in patients with a petrous apex lesion.[1] Pain in the distribution of the ipsilateral trigeminal nerve in the presence of a petrous apex mass can be explained by compression or irritation of the cisternal segment or the Gausserian ganglion and is seen in approximately 20% of patients with cholesterol granuloma.[8] Double vision is occasionally identified and results from compression of the sixth nerve in Dorello canal. Facial spasm/weakness results from irritation or compression of the seventh nerve in the internal auditory canal, cerebellopontine angle, or the fallopian canal and occurs in up to 20% of patients with petrous apex cholesterol granuloma.[8] Sensorineural hearing loss, ear fullness, tinnitus (65%), and dizziness (50%) from compression of the eighth nerve or erosion into the otic capsule are seen with involvement of the internal auditory canal or lateral extension of petrous apex cholesterol granuloma.[8] Dysphagia, hoarseness, and shoulder pain/weakness are rarely seen with aggressive malignancies originating in the petrous apex such as chordoma, chondrosarcoma, or metastatic disease. Unilateral serous otitis media is sometimes identified with petrous apex lesions, which compress or erode into the eustachian tube.

EVALUATION AND DIAGNOSIS

A complete history and physical examination are standard parts of the evaluation of any patient with complex skull base pathology. A thorough examination of the cranial nerves, with attention to ocular motility, facial function, hearing, balance, and facial sensation, is of paramount importance. Otoscopy can sometimes reveal a unilateral effusion or retrotympanic mass depending on the extent of the lesion. Tuning fork examination provides basic information on the presence of sensorineural or conductive hearing loss and confirms the results of audiometry. A head impulse test is a simple and rapid way to assess for a vestibular deficit involving the lateral semicircular canal.[9]

Pure tone and speech audiometry provides objective information on the extent of middle ear and eighth nerve involvement. The audiogram is critically important when selecting a surgical approach in the event that management of the petrous apex lesion is required.

Radiographic studies are the single most important diagnostic modality. The differential diagnosis and radiographic features for petrous apex lesions include a variety of inflammatory and neoplastic conditions (**Table 1**). Imaging also assists with determining a potential surgical approach in the event operative management is required. Computed tomography (CT) provides a detailed view of the osseous anatomy of the skull base. Structures readily defined by CT include the otic capsule, carotid canal, jugular foramen, fallopian canal, semicanal of the tensor tympani muscle, eustachian tube, and all of the foramina within the skull base. CT allows for delineation of a petrous apex lesion relative to adjacent structures within the temporal bone. Intralesional calcifications are also easily visualized on CT and can help narrow the differential diagnosis. Surgical access to a petrous apex lesion is often determined using CT and can also be used for image guidance at the time of the procedure. Petrous apex cholesterol granulomas demonstrate smooth erosion of the petrous apex.[10] Erosion into the internal auditory canal, otic capsule, fallopian canal, petrous carotid canal, jugular foramen, or outside the confines of the petrous apex is readily demonstrated on CT (**Fig. 1**). CT angiography/venography is sometimes necessary in cases in which the cholesterol granuloma has eroded into the carotid canal or jugular foramen with resultant vascular compression (**Fig. 2**). CT angiography/venography provides critical information on surgical access relative to the distorted vascular anatomy.[11] CT is also sometimes utilized to follow patients who are asymptomatic or who have undergone surgical management to monitor for recurrence or progression. Aeration of the petrous apex after surgical management has not been shown to correlate with recurrence.[12]

MRI has allowed for significant advances in the diagnosis and management of skull base pathology. MRI significantly narrows the differential diagnosis of a petrous apex

Table 1
Differential diagnosis and radiographic characteristics of petrous apex lesions

Lesion	MRI				CT	Other
	T1 Without Gadolinium	T1 With Gadolinium	T1 Fat Saturated Gadolinium	T2		
Cholesterol granuloma	Hyperintense	No enhancement	No enhancement	Hyperintense	Smooth erosion	
Petrous apicitis	Hypointense	Rim enhancement	Rim enhancement	Hyperintense	Destroyed septae and possible cortex	
CSF cyst/cephalocele	Hypointense	No enhancement	No enhancement	Hyperintense	Smooth erosion	May connect to Meckel cave No restricted diffusion on diffusion weighted imaging
Epidermoid	Hypointense	No enhancement	No enhancement	Hyperintense	Smooth erosion	Restricted diffusion on diffusion weighted imaging
Effusion	Iso- to hypointense	Slight enhancement	Slight enhancement	Hyperintense	Intact septation	Hyperintense on FLAIR
Mucocele	Isointense	No enhancement	No enhancement	Hyperintense	Destroyed septae	
Asymmetric pneumatization	Hyperintense	No enhancement	Hypointense, no enhancement	Hypointense	Marrow on lesion side, air cells contralateral side	
Carotid aneurysm	New thrombus–hypointense, Old thrombus–hyperintense			Hyperintense	Smooth expansion of carotid canal, heterogeneous contrast enhancement	MRI–central flow void, onion skin appearance

Chordoma	Hypo- to isointense	Enhancement less intense than chondrosarcoma	Enhancement	Hyperintense	Lobulated, bone destruction with residual fragments	Centrally located in clivus with lateral spread to petrous apex
Chondrosarcoma	Hypo- to isointense	Enhancement	Enhancement	Hyperintense, heterogeneous	Infiltrative, remnants of eroded bone	Centered in petrous apex in region of foramen lacerum, calcified areas may show as signal voids
Metastasis	Depends on primary	Enhancement	Enhancement	Depends on primary	Bone erosion	
Paraganglioma	Isointense	Enhancement, flow voids	Enhancement, flow voids	Hyperintense	Opacified and destroyed air cells	Vascular blush on angio
Meningioma	Iso- to hypointense	Enhancement	Enhancement	Iso- to hyperintense	Hyperostosis, Iso- or hyperdense calcifications	Dural tails, sessile–broad interface with bone or tentorium
Schwannoma	Isointense	Enhancement	Enhancement	Hyper- or Hypointense	May show dilation of internal auditory canal	Centered over porus acousticus
Plasmacytoma	Isointense	Enhancement	Enhancement	Hypointense	Irregular to smooth bone erosion	Fluorodeoxygluocos PET enhancement
Vascular malformation	Intermediate	Enhancement	Enhancement	Heterogeneous hyperintense	Destruction of osseous septae	

Data from Refs. [1,10,35–39]; and Adapted from Isaacson B, Kutz JW, Roland PS. Lesions of the petrous apex: diagnosis and management. Otolaryngol Clin North Am 2007;40(3):482–483; with permission.

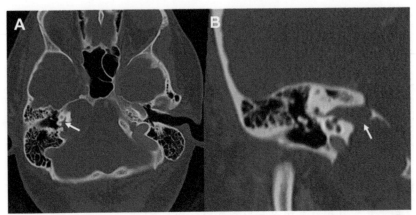

Fig. 1. (*A*) Axial bone window CT scan demonstrating a right petrous apex cholesterol granuloma with erosion into the medial aspect of the inferior basal turn of the cochlea (*arrow*). (*B*) Coronal bone window CT scan demonstrating a right petrous apex cholesterol granuloma with erosion into the inferior aspect of the internal auditory canal (*arrow*).

lesion, thus obviating the need for obtaining tissue to establish a diagnosis in most cases. MRI is often used in patients undergoing observation of an asymptomatic petrous apex lesion and can readily identify disease progression. Cholesterol granuloma is hyperintense on T1 and T2 MRI images, which readily distinguish it from other lesions of the petrous apex (**Fig. 3**). A heterogeneous signal is often seen on MRI with cholesterol granuloma, which often represents fragments of bone and the solid material that is seen within these lesions. Extraosseous extension of a cholesterol

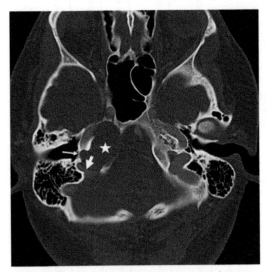

Fig. 2. Axial bone window CT venogram demonstrates a right petrous apex cholesterol granuloma (*star*) with significant carotid canal and jugular foramen erosion. Posterior compression of the jugular bulb by the cholesterol granuloma is demonstrated (*large arrow*). The infracochlear tract (*small arrow*) is available for marsupialization of the cholesterol granuloma into the middle ear.

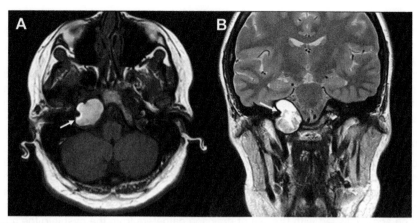

Fig. 3. (*A*) Axial T1 MRI without gadolinium demonstrates a hyperintense large right petrous apex lesion (*arrow*) consistent with a cholesterol granuloma. (*B*) A coronal T2 MRI image demonstrates a large hyperintense right petrous apex mass (*arrow*) consistent with a petrous apex cholesterol granuloma.

granuloma is also better visualized with MRI as opposed to CT, although both techniques are complementary.[10] Conventional angiography is sometimes utilized to determine tumor vascularity and in some cases for embolization to reduce intraoperative bleeding in patients with vascular lesions.[1]

MANAGEMENT

Observation with serial imaging is the most appropriate management in patients with incidentally discovered asymptomatic petrous apex cholesterol granulomas. Sudden onset of new symptoms related to rapid enlargement of a petrous apex cholesterol granuloma has been reported.[13] MRI is often used to follow these lesions given the absence of radiation exposure and better soft tissue resolution compared with CT. The administration of gadolinium on follow-up examinations is unnecessary once the diagnosis has been established as the cholesterol granulomas are already hyperintense on T1 images. CT is often used in subjects who cannot tolerate an MRI examination or in patients who have pacemakers or other ferromagnetic implants. CT has the advantage of being a less expensive study and having the ability to obtain images rapidly.[14]

Surgical management of cholesterol granulomas is recommended in symptomatic patients or those with impending complications (eg, hearing loss and vestibular symptoms from otic capsule erosion). Several approaches have been described to access the petrous apex, and these can generally be classified as transtemporal or transnasal, as well as those that preserve hearing and those that do not preserve hearing. Surgical management entails either excision or marsupialization of the cholesterol granuloma. Cholesterol granuloma excision usually requires wide exposure of the lesion and often necessitates a craniotomy with associated brain retraction. Advantages of excision are the potential for reducing recurrence. Disadvantages include the need for brain retraction, which can result in encephalomalacia and rarely seizures, and increased risk of postoperative intracranial hemorrhage. Cerebrospinal fluid (CSF) leakage is also a risk of intracranial procedures, especially in patients with cholesterol granuloma, who often have hyperpneumatized temporal bones. Craniotomy approaches often necessitate a longer hospital stay to assess for potential intracranial complications. Marsupialization by creation of a wide drainage tract into a mucosalized space often allows decompression of an expanding symptomatic cholesterol granuloma. Most marsupialization approaches do not require a craniotomy, and in some cases they can be performed as an outpatient procedure. CSF leaks are occasionally seen with these approaches. A significant disadvantage of marsupialization is recurrence of symptoms secondary to cicatrix obstructing the surgically created drainage tract.[1,15]

Extradural Middle Fossa Approach

Excision or marsupialization of a petrous apex cholesterol granuloma can be accomplished with an extradural middle fossa subtemporal approach. Complete excision of the lesion with apical obliteration with fat or other materials potentially reduces the chance of recurrence.[16] Marsupialization via a middle fossa approach can be accomplished with the use of drainage catheters from the cyst into the mastoid. Maintenance of catheter patency is often challenging, resulting in progression of the cholesterol granuloma. Kamiguchi and colleagues[17] described an alternative method of drainage by drilling a tract between the petrous apex cholesterol into the anterior epitympanic space. The greater superficial petrosal nerve is identified, and drilling is commenced medial to this structure just anterior to the cochlea. The tract is then extended into the anterior epitympanic recess above the tensor tympani muscle. A dehiscent petrous carotid artery in some cases may not permit creation of this drainage pathway.[17]

Hearing Preservation Transtemporal Approaches

The infra- or subcochlear approach, initially described by Ghorayeb and Jahrsdoerfer, utilizes a postauricular transcanal exposure to access the petrous apex.[18] A superiorly based tympanomeatal flap is elevated, and the medial inferior tympanic bone, along with the osseous annulus, is carefully lowered to the level of the floor of the hypotympanum. Intraoperative facial nerve monitoring is beneficial, as the vertical facial nerve closely approximates the posterior inferior osseous annulus and can be exposed or injured as the inferior osseous canal is expanded. The osseous wall of inferior basal turn of the cochlea, jugular bulb, and the petrous carotid artery are the key landmarks that are exposed and identified within the medial wall of the meso- and hypotympanum. Occasionally larger or more laterally based cholesterol granulomas present to the lateral aspect of the infracochlear tract and can readily be exteriorized into the middle ear with minimal bone removal. Medially located cholesterol granulomas require more extensive drilling, which can sometimes be limited by a large jugular bulb, or a posteriorly positioned petrous carotid artery. A wide opening is created in the thick wall of the cholesterol granuloma in order to reduce the chance of postoperative obstruction.[18] The mean dimensions of this approach, in a study of 20 cadaveric specimens, were 9.41 mm by 7.33 mm.[19] Placement of stents does not seem to alter the natural history of tract obstruction.[12] CSF leaks can also be encountered if the angle of drilling is directed posteriorly toward the posterior fossa dura and cochlear aqueduct. Tympanic membrane perforation is also a risk of this approach, which may occur if there is a tear in the tympanomeatal flap at the time of elevation or with drilling. Hearing loss and vertigo can occur if there is violation of the otic capsule or if the vein of the cochlear aqueduct is injured. Venous bleeding from the jugular bulb can typically be controlled with gentle compression with resorbable packing material and cotton. Carotid artery injury is rare but requires emergent interventional angiography.[16]

The transcanal endoscopic infracochlear approach provides a new minimally invasive procedure for management of petrous apex cholesterol granulomas. The endoscope provides a wide-angle view as opposed to the line-of-site view seen with the microscope. The ear canal is used a surgical corridor as opposed to a post-auricular incision. A wide superior-based tympanomeatal flap is also utilized for access similar to the traditional postauricular transcanal infracochlear approach. The petrous carotid artery, jugular bulb, and inferior cochlear basal turn are the limits of the dissection, which proceeds medially until the wall of cholesterol granuloma is identified and opened. Advantages of this approach include reduced intraoperative bleeding, wide-angle view, and the ability to provide a view within the cholesterol granuloma to remove loculations.[20,21] Postoperative pain is also decreased, as only ear canal incisions are necessary. Disadvantages of this technique include using 1 hand for instrumentation, as the other hand is used to hold the scope, loss of depth of field, and difficulty controlling bleeding.[21]

The infralabyrinthine approach utilizes a postauricular transmastoid exposure to marsupialize a cholesterol granuloma. A complete mastoidectomy is performed in addition to identification of the posterior semicircular canal, sigmoid sinus, jugular bulb, and vertical facial nerve. A wide opening is created in the wall of the cholesterol granuloma in order to reduce the chance of tract obstruction. The mean dimensions of the infralabyrinthine approach in 20 cadaveric specimens were 4.99 mm by 7.23 mm.[19] In Habercamp's study, 8 out of the 20 petrous apices were inaccessible via the infralabyrinthine approach secondary to a high jugular bulb.[19] CSF leak can also be seen, especially if the drill is angled posteriorly into the posterior fossa dura.[22] Vertigo and hearing loss may occur if the posterior semicircular canal is violated or if the vein of the cochlear aqueduct is injured.

The subarcuate, sinodural angle, and supracochlear approaches all provide narrow access to the petrous apex and are usually used for the management of acute petrositis.[2] All of these approaches utilize a postauricular transmastoid exposure. The subarcuate approach requires skeletonization of the semicircular canals. A 2 mm diamond is used to open the space inferior to the arch of the superior canal and superior to the vestibule. The mean diameter of this approach in the anterior–posterior dimension is 4.88 mm, and the mean diameter in the superior inferior dimension is 4.9 mm. This tract can be followed to the posterior superior petrous apex. These dimensions were noted to be increased in cadaveric temporal bones with aeration along the subarcuate track.[23] Vestibular dysfunction and hearing loss are significant risks secondary to violation of the otic capsule with the subarcuate approach.[23] The sinodural angle approach entails skeletonization of the semicircular canals and middle and posterior fossa dura. The area between the middle and posterior fossa plates and the semicircular canals is followed medially into the posterior superior petrous apex. Vestibular dysfunction and hearing loss are significant risks secondary to violation of the otic capsule with the subarcuate approach. The supracochlear approach necessitates opening the zygomatic root air cells and usually requires removal of the incus and possibly the malleus head. The anterior aspect of the superior semicircular canal, tegmen tympani, and tympanic facial nerve serve as the limits of the supracochlear approach. Drilling commences anterior to the superior semicircular canal, and between the tegmen tympani and the tympanic facial nerve to access the anterior superior petrous apex. The mean size of this opening on anatomic dissections was 7 mm between the superior semicircular canal and the geniculate ganglion along the tegmen, 5.3 mm from superior semicircular canal to the geniculate ganglion along the fallopian canal, and 4.8 mm from the tympanic fallopian canal to the tegmen tympani along the anterior wall of the superior semicircular canal.[24] The labyrinthine facial nerve may be injured while using the supracochlear approach, making facial nerve monitoring indispensable. Vestibular dysfunction and CSF leak are also a risk of this approach, resulting from violation of the superior semicircular canal and the middle fossa dura respectively.[2,24,25]

Nonhearing Transtemporal Approaches

Patients with symptomatic petrous apex cholesterol granuloma with nonserviceable hearing can be managed with either a transotic or a translabyrinthine approach. Long-standing hearing loss should be a prerequisite for these approaches. Rihani and colleagues recently demonstrated reversible sensorineural hearing loss in 2 patients with cholesterol granuloma invading the otic capsule after undergoing an infracochlear approach. Posterior petrous apex cholesterol granulomas with poor residual hearing can be managed with a translabyrinthine approach. This postauricular transmastoid approach entails removal of the semicircular canals and vestibule and identification of the internal auditory canal. This approach provides limited access to the anterior petrous apex. Risks of this procedure include CSF leak, facial nerve injury, vestibular dysfunction, and loss of residual hearing. The transotic approach provides access to the entire petrous apex. This approach utilizes the same steps as the translabyrinthine approach, with the addition of overclosure of the ear canal with removal of the posterior canal wall as well as the cochlea. The facial nerve is left in the fallopian canal with the transotic approach as opposed the transcochlear approach, where the entire intratemporal portion of the nerve is rerouted posteriorly. The transotic approach has the same risks as the translabyrinthine approach in addition to carotid artery injury, and iatrogenic cholesteatoma from incomplete removal of skin from the external auditory canal. The transotic and transcochlear approaches usually require obliteration of the eustachian tube, as CSF leakage is often encountered at the time the cochlectomy. These approaches allow for marsupialization and in some cases complete excision of the facial nerve.[8]

Transnasal Endoscopic Approach

The transnasal endoscopic approach can, in select cases, provide a wide drainage tract in patients with a petrous apex cholesterol granuloma. This approach typically requires a wide sphenoidotomy with creation of a large tract into the lesion, usually along the posterior lateral wall of the sphenoid sinus. Identification and in some cases mobilization of the petrous carotid artery can be performed in lesions that do not present along the posterior lateral wall of the sphenoid sinus. This approach requires a wide maxillary antrostomy and complete ethmoidectomy in addition to removal of the posterior wall of the maxillary sinus to expose the pterygomaxillary fissure and infratemporal fossa. The petrous carotid artery is identified, and a drainage tract is then created from the sinus cavity into the petrous apex cholesterol granuloma. This approach has several advantages over the transtemporal approach, including being an incisionless procedure. A substantially larger drainage tract can typically be created with a transnasal approach, which is less likely to close with scar. Removal of scar tissue to reestablish drainage may be performed in the clinic in some cases. Risks of this approach include epistaxis, CSF leak, dry nose, eye injury, brain injury, carotid artery injury, and facial anesthesia.[26,27]

OUTCOMES AND PROGNOSIS

The primary end point for management of petrous apex cholesterol granuloma is resolution or improvement of presenting symptoms. A recent systematic review of the endonasal approach for management of petrous apex cholesterol granuloma demonstrated that 84.4% of 45 patients experienced resolution of presenting symptoms, while an additional 13.3% of patients experienced improvement. Restenosis of the drainage pathway was noted in 9 of 45 (20%) patients in this review; however, only 4 of these 9 patients with recurrent stenosis were symptomatic. There was no difference in recurrence rate with or without stent placement in this review. The complication rate was 13.3% with the endoscopic approach, which included epistaxis, chronic serous otitis media requiring tympanostomy tube placement, chronic sphenoid sinusitis, and transient sixth nerve palsy. One patient experienced several major complications including clival venous hemorrhage requiring transfusion, CSF leak, tension pneumocephalus, diplopia, unilateral leg weakness, nystagmus, and severe headaches that resolved with conservative measures.[15]

A review of 79 open or transtemporal approaches revealed 71 of 79 (90%) patients experienced symptom resolution, with an overall recurrence rate of 12.5%. The complication rate of open procedures was 24.3% and ranged from 0% to 60%. The most common complications seen in open approaches were hearing loss and CSF leak. Hearing loss occurred in anywhere between 3% and 83% of patients depending on which series was reviewed. A nonhearing preservation approach was used in several of the studies reporting a higher hearing loss rate. Transient facial paralysis was also seen in up to 30% of patients in several series. Severe complications were rare but significant, including seizures, meningitis, internal carotid artery hemorrhage, and internal carotid artery occlusion with subsequent mortality.[8,15,16,28–34]

SUMMARY

Petrous apex cholesterol granuloma is a unique inflammatory process that can present with similar symptoms and signs as neoplastic disease. Marsupialization through a variety of approaches often results in resolution or improvement of presenting symptoms. Image guidance and minimally invasive transnasal approaches are some of the more recent advances in the management of petrous apex cholesterol granuloma.

REFERENCES

1. Isaacson B, Kutz JW, Roland PS. Lesions of the petrous apex: diagnosis and management. Otolaryngol Clin North Am 2007;40(3):479–519, viii.
2. Chole RA. Petrous apicitis: surgical anatomy. Ann Otol Rhinol Laryngol 1985; 94(3):251–7.
3. Arriaga MA. Petrous apex effusion: a clinical disorder. Laryngoscope 2006; 116(8):1349–56.
4. Lo WW, Solti-Bohman LG, Brackmann DE, et al. Cholesterol granuloma of the petrous apex: CT diagnosis. Radiology 1984;153(3):705–11.
5. Arriaga MA, Brackmann DE. Differential diagnosis of primary petrous apex lesions. Am J Otol 1991;12(6):470–4.
6. Jackler RK, Cho M. A new theory to explain the genesis of petrous apex cholesterol granuloma. Otol Neurotol 2003;24(1):96–106 [discussion: 106].
7. Hoa M, House JW, Linthicum FH Jr. Petrous apex cholesterol granuloma: maintenance of drainage pathway, the histopathology of surgical management and histopathologic evidence for the exposed marrow theory. Otol Neurotol 2012; 33(6):1059–65.
8. Brackmann DE, Toh EH. Surgical management of petrous apex cholesterol granulomas. Otol Neurotol 2002;23(4):529–33.

9. Halmagyi GM, Curthoys IS. A clinical sign of canal paresis. Arch Neurol 1988; 45(7):737–9.
10. Chang P, Fagan PA, Atlas MD, et al. Imaging destructive lesions of the petrous apex. Laryngoscope 1998;108(4 Pt 1):599–604.
11. Isaacson B, Kutz JW Jr, Mendelsohn D, et al. CT venography: use in selecting a surgical approach for the treatment of petrous apex cholesterol granulomas. Otol Neurotol 2009;30(3):386–91.
12. Castillo MP, Samy RN, Isaacson B, et al. Petrous apex cholesterol granuloma aeration: does it matter? Otolaryngol Head Neck Surg 2008;138(4):518–22.
13. Thorne MC, Gebarski SS, Telian SA. Rapid expansion in a previously indolent cholesterol cyst: a need for lifelong follow-up. Otol Neurotol 2006;27(1):124–6.
14. Moore KR, Harnsberger HR, Shelton C, et al. "Leave me alone" lesions of the petrous apex. AJNR Am J Neuroradiol 1998;19(4):733–8.
15. Eytan DF, Kshettry VR, Sindwani R, et al. Surgical outcomes after endoscopic management of cholesterol granulomas of the petrous apex: a systematic review. Neurosurg Focus 2014;37(4):E14.
16. Kusumi M, Fukushima T, Mehta AI, et al. Middle fossa approach for total resection of petrous apex cholesterol granulomas: use of vascularized galeofascial flap preventing recurrence. Neurosurgery 2013;72(1 Suppl Operative):77–86 [discussion: 86].
17. Kamiguchi H, Kawase T, Toya S, et al. Cholesterol granuloma of the petrous apex: establishment of a drainage route into the superior tympanic cavity–technical note. Neurol Med Chir (Tokyo) 1996;36(9):662–5.
18. Ghorayeb BY, Jahrsdoerfer RA. Subcochlear approach for cholesterol granulomas of the inferior petrous apex. Otolaryngol Head Neck Surg 1990;103(1):60–5.
19. Haberkamp TJ. Surgical anatomy of the transtemporal approaches to the petrous apex. Am J Otol 1997;18(4):501–6.
20. Mattox DE. Endoscopy-assisted surgery of the petrous apex. Otolaryngol Head Neck Surg 2004;130(2):229–41.
21. Presutti L, Nogueira JF, Alicandri-Ciufelli M, et al. Beyond the middle ear: endoscopic surgical anatomy and approaches to inner ear and lateral skull base. Otolaryngol Clin North Am 2013;46(2):189–200.
22. Comert E, Comert A, Cay N, et al. Surgical anatomy of the infralabyrinthine approach. Otolaryngol Head Neck Surg 2014;151(2):301–7.
23. Lee A, Hamidi S, Djalilian H. Anatomy of the transarcuate approach to the petrous apex. Otolaryngol Head Neck Surg 2009;140(6):880–3.
24. Telischi FF, Luntz M, Whiteman ML. Supracochlear approach to the petrous apex: case report and anatomic study. Am J Otol 1999;20(4):500–4.
25. Gerek M, Satar B, Yazar F, et al. Transcanal anterior approach for cystic lesions of the petrous apex. Otol Neurotol 2004;25(6):973–6.
26. Griffith AJ, Terrell JE. Transsphenoid endoscopic management of petrous apex cholesterol granuloma. Otolaryngol Head Neck Surg 1996;114(1):91–4.
27. Fucci MJ, Alford EL, Lowry LD, et al. Endoscopic management of a giant cholesterol cyst of the petrous apex. Skull Base Surg 1994;4(1):52–8.
28. Thedinger BA, Nadol JB Jr, Montgomery WW, et al. Radiographic diagnosis, surgical treatment, and long-term follow-up of cholesterol granulomas of the petrous apex. Laryngoscope 1989;99(9):896–907.
29. Goldofsky E, Hoffman RA, Holliday RA, et al. Cholesterol cysts of the temporal bone: diagnosis and treatment. Ann Otol Rhinol Laryngol 1991;100(3):181–7.
30. Brodkey JA, Robertson JH, Shea JJ 3rd, et al. Cholesterol granulomas of the petrous apex: combined neurosurgical and otological management. J Neurosurg 1996;85(4):625–33.

31. Eisenberg MB, Haddad G, Al-Mefty O. Petrous apex cholesterol granulomas: evolution and management. J Neurosurg 1997;86(5):822–9.
32. Mosnier I, Cyna-Gorse F, Grayeli AB, et al. Management of cholesterol granulomas of the petrous apex based on clinical and radiologic evaluation. Otol Neurotol 2002;23(4):522–8.
33. Sanna M, Dispenza F, Mathur N, et al. Otoneurological management of petrous apex cholesterol granuloma. Am J Otolaryngol 2009;30(6):407–14.
34. Cristante L, Puchner MA. A keyhole middle fossa approach to large cholesterol granulomas of the petrous apex. Surg Neurol 2000;53(1):64–70 [discussion: 70–1].
35. Sanna M, Zini C, Gamoletti R, et al. Petrous bone cholesteatoma. Skull Base Surg 1993;3(4):201–13.
36. Moore KR, Fischbein NJ, Harnsberger HR, et al. Petrous apex cephaloceles. AJNR Am J Neuroradiol 2001;22(10):1867–71.
37. Frank E, Brown BM, Wilson DF. Asymptomatic fusiform aneurysm of the petrous carotid artery in a patient with von Recklinghausen's neurofibromatosis. Surg Neurol 1989;32(1):75–8.
38. Purcell P, Isaacson B, Oliver DH, et al. Petrous apex vascular malformation. Otol Neurotol 2012;33(8):e67–8.
39. Cistaro A, Durando S, Paze F, et al. Expansive masses arising from the clivus: the role Of FDG-PET/CT in the metabolic assessment of skeletal lesions. J Radiol Case Rep 2009;3(11):33–40.

Rhabdomyosarcoma and Other Pediatric Temporal Bone Malignancies

Michael B. Gluth, MD

KEYWORDS

- Rhabdomyosarcoma • Ear • Temporal bone • Sarcoma • Carcinoma

KEY POINTS

- In children, sarcomas are the most common malignant tumors affecting the ear and temporal bone, with rhabdomyosarcoma (RMS) being the most frequently encountered.
- The formalized assessment of RMS involves assigning a tumor stage and then determining a surgical-histopathologic grouping; these, alongside tumor histology, determine a patient's risk group classification, prognosis, and further treatment.
- The ideal treatment of localized RMS includes complete surgical resection followed by chemotherapy and radiation therapy; however, gross total resection is not always possible because of the associated risk and morbidity depending on which structures are invaded.
- Typical RMS of the temporal bone without distant metastasis usually falls in the low- or intermediate-risk classification; the determining whether low- or intermediate-risk group should be assigned generally hinges on whether or not gross (not microscopic) tumor removal is achieved.

INTRODUCTION

Malignancy of the ear and temporal bone in the pediatric population is a complex and challenging problem for many reasons. Cancer in children evokes a particular energy that supercharges emotions; thus, attending to these patients requires an extra measure of empathy, professionalism, and objectivity. In addition, malignant tumors of the ear and temporal bone are extraordinarily uncommon in children, rendering clinical decision making difficult. It is often necessary to infer best practice from outcomes reported for the management of these tumors treated in other parts of the body or for similar tumors occurring in adults. Reliance on the expertise of other oncologic

No conflict of interest of funding source to disclose.
Bloom Otopathology Laboratory, Section of Otolaryngology–Head & Neck Surgery, Comprehensive Ear & Hearing Center, University of Chicago Medicine & Biological Sciences, MC 1035, 5841 South Maryland Avenue, Chicago, IL 60637, USA
E-mail address: mgluth1@surgery.bsd.uchicago.edu

Otolaryngol Clin N Am 48 (2015) 375–390
http://dx.doi.org/10.1016/j.otc.2014.12.010
0030-6665/15/$ – see front matter © 2015 Elsevier Inc. All rights reserved.

Abbreviations	
ARMS	Alveolar rhabdomyosarcoma
COG-STS	Soft Tissue Sarcoma Committee of the Children's Oncology Group
CT	Computed tomography
ERMS	Embryonal rhabdomyosarcoma
LCH	Langerhans cell histiocytosis
LTBR	Lateral temporal bone resection
MRI	Magnetic resonance imaging
NRMSS	Nonrhabdomyosarcomatous sarcoma
RMS	Rhabdomyosarcoma
STBR	Subtotal temporal bone resection

specialists and the need for periodic review of the pertinent medical literature is expected when an obscure tumor is at hand because it would be rare in the career of a skull base surgeon to ever develop a working familiarity and comfort with all the various forms of cancer that can potentially involve the ear and temporal bone of a child. Therefore, this article provides an overview of some of the malignant tumors of the ear and temporal bone that occur in children with a particular emphasis on RMS. In addition, it outlines the key principles of evaluation and management that have particular relevance to the pediatric perspective.

PRESENTATION

With a few caveats, the presentation of ear and temporal bone malignancy in children is similar to what is encountered in adults.[1,2] Classically, these tumors mimic a severe and refractory ear infection. The most common presenting symptoms and signs are hearing loss, otorrhea, otalgia, headache, aural polyp, facial nerve weakness, and regional lymphadenopathy. However, unlike adult patients, children may be less apt to verbalize the presence of hearing loss and will typically have been treated for infection for a much longer period of time before the possibility of malignancy is considered. Also, it is important to recognize that children with cancer generally begin to lose weight and fail to thrive at an earlier stage than adults, especially very young children.

Assessment of neurologic function in affected children may reveal various cranial nerve deficits. Ophthalmic abnormalities such as visual loss, diplopia, proptosis, and chemosis are ominous indicators of a combined lateral and anterior skull base tumor with potential involvement of the cavernous sinus and orbital apex. Yet, diplopia due to isolated weakness of the sixth cranial nerve can be encountered in less-extensive temporal bone tumors that involve the petrous apex while still being confined to the base of the middle cranial fossa. Similarly, isolated numbness in the distribution of the mandibular branch of the fifth cranial nerve may be an indicator that tumor involves the lateral skull base in the infratemporal fossa without an extensive anterior skull base component. Indicators of lower cranial nerve dysfunction such as glottic insufficiency, dysphagia, shoulder weakness, or tongue weakness on the affected side suggest tumor invasion of the jugular foramen or hypoglossal canal. However, for a slow-growing tumor, symptoms of lower cranial neuropathy may be subtle because a child's capacity to rapidly adapt and compensate can be surprisingly robust.

Depending on the extent and location of a malignant tumor in the temporal bone, other presenting signs and symptoms are possible. Trismus or pain with chewing may indicate tumor involvement of the temporomandibular joint or supporting muscles of mastication. Vertigo or imbalance may signify invasion of the labyrinth or vestibular nerve. In cases in which the ear and temporal bone are invaded secondarily, primary tumor of the parotid gland, pharynx, mandible, or upper cervical structures may be evident. Invasion of the dura or brain should be considered when cerebrospinal fluid leakage or a recent history of meningitis is present. Finally, obstruction of the sigmoid sinus or jugular bulb because of tumor bulk or direct invasion may infrequently cause symptoms of central venous congestion ranging from headache to cerebral edema.

EVALUATION AND DIAGNOSIS

Keeping the above-described signs and symptoms in mind, a detailed history is taken, and a complete head and neck examination that includes microotoscopy is performed. Audiologic testing is also undertaken to document hearing thresholds. When skull base disease process is suspected, the next diagnostic step is radiologic imaging. As this may be difficult to obtain in children, general anesthesia is a common requirement, and it is therefore ideal to complete all required testing at once, which in the case of a skull base tumor usually means acquisition of contrasted magnetic resonance imaging (MRI) and computed tomography (CT) in the same setting. Sometimes it is also possible to complete a soft tissue biopsy while the child is under anesthesia when tumor is evident on examination in an easily accessible location.

Evaluation of skull base disease relies heavily on radiologic imaging, and both MRI and CT are complementary in portraying a tumor's characteristics and extent. Typical imaging characteristics of various malignant skull base lesions are portrayed in **Table 1**.

One aspect unique in the assessment of pediatric ear and temporal bone malignancy that deserves mention is the need to differentiate cancer from Langerhans cell histiocytosis (LCH), a pseudomalignant process often encountered in children that may share several presenting features with malignant tumors such as chronic otorrhea, otalgia, headache, lymphadenopathy, and hearing loss.[3] LCH (previously known as histiocytosis X) is a rare locally destructive condition that involves clonal proliferation of Langerhans cells, which in turn may migrate from skin to regional lymph nodes. LCH is considered a pseudomalignancy because many cases of spontaneous remission have been reported and also because much of the associated pathophysiology seems to be related to local cytokine-mediated reactive processes. Langerhans cells, which resemble epidermal dendritic cells, group together with lymphocytes and eosinophils to generate destructive inflammatory lesions, which can occur anywhere in the body. Diagnosis of LCH is strongly supported by the typical histopathologic appearance and positive immunohistologic staining for CD1a antigen, S-100, adenosine triphosphatase, and mannosidase. Definitive diagnosis is confirmed by the presence of Birbeck granules in the cytoplasm of affected Langerhans cells, which are evident on electron microscopy.[4]

TREATMENT
Microsurgery

The decision to perform microsurgical resection of a malignant tumor from the ear and temporal bone of a child is made thoughtfully and is based on input from a variety of pediatric specialties including medical oncology, radiation oncology, otolaryngology, anesthesiology, neurosurgery, and facial plastic surgery. Choice of a particular surgical approach should be individualized based on a child's tumor specifics (subtype, involved structures, stage) and tolerance of relevant surgical morbidity. It is critical that the patient, family, and treatment team are collectively in agreement with the

Table 1
Imaging characteristics of various malignant temporal bone tumors

Lesion	MRI			CT
	T1	T1 + Gd	T2	
Rhabdomyosarcoma	Hypointense/isointense	Enhancement	Hyperintense	Destructive, infiltrative
Fibrosarcoma	Hypointense	Strong enhancement	Hyperintense	Expansile with calcification
Ewing sarcoma	Hypointense	No enhancement	Mixed	Well circumscribed with hyperostosis
Osteosarcoma	Irregular hypointense/ isointense	Irregular enhancement	Mixed	Radiolucent
Chloroma	Hypointense	Enhancement	Isointense	Expansile, homogeneous
Squamous cell carcinoma	Isointense	Enhancement	Hyperintense	Destructive, invasive
Chordoma	Hypointense/isointense	Enhancement	Hyperintense	Lobulated, bony destruction with bony spicules
Chondrosarcoma	Hypointense/isointense	Enhancement	Hyperintense	Infiltrative bony destruction with bony spicules
Parotid mucoepidermoid carcinoma	Hypintense, especially in cystic spaces	Irregular enhancement of solid components	Hypointense/isointense	Poorly defined border, cystic spaces
Metastasis	Variable	Enhancement	Variable	Bony erosion
Lymphoma	Hypointense	Variable, higher grade will enhance	Isointense	Irregular with smooth margins

Abbreviation: Gd, gadolinium.

goals and intended degree of aggressiveness of surgery, which may range from wide resection with curative intent to diagnostic soft tissue biopsy. If the projected morbidity of a planned surgical resection involves significant disfigurement, it is critically important to initiate early child and adult psychiatric consultations for support of the patient, siblings, and other family members. In addition, utilization of a child life specialist during periods of inpatient hospitalization may help the patient cope with fear and discomfort.

Although lateral skull base surgery in adults and in children is based on similar anatomic principles, there are a few particular considerations in children worth noting.[5] First, because of future projected growth of a child's craniofacial skeleton, it may be desirable to favor craniofacial plates that resorb if any are deemed necessary.[6] Metallic plates not only have the potential to distort future radiologic imaging but also tend to progressively migrate into the inner table of the skull over time. Second, a young child's tolerance of heavy blood loss is considerably less than that of an adult. This fact is particularly relevant if the surgeon intends to pursue tumor into the jugular foramen, where robust bleeding is commonplace. Thus, the decision to dissect tumor away from any of the great vessels should always be made cautiously and with appropriate preoperative preparation such as vascular imaging, blood products on immediate standby, interventional radiology availability, and proactive availability of relevant surgical materials (eg, Fogarty catheters, thrombin-soaked absorbable packing, vessel loops). Last, it should be kept in mind that a child's tolerance of complex postoperative wound care is typically much less than what would be expected for an adult. Thus, reconstructive techniques that allow complete closure of the surgical wound and primary closure of the donor site, such as the anterolateral thigh free flap, are favored over techniques that might require repetitive ear cleaning or dressing changes such as a split thickness skin graft.[7]

Although a comprehensive review of all microsurgical skull base approaches that can be used to approach a child's temporal bone malignancy is not intended, a general subdivision and discussion of the most commonly used techniques for malignant temporal bone tumors is summarized in the discussion that follows.

Temporal bone resection

Tumors primarily originating from the ear canal or tympanomastoid compartment are generally managed with some type of temporal bone resection.[8] The most common form of this procedure and the only one that affords the possibility of en bloc tumor removal is lateral temporal bone resection (LTBR), which involves radical resection of the entire ear canal (bony and membranous), tympanic membrane, and underlying malleus manubrium in a single self-contained specimen (**Fig. 1**). Extensive tumors that invade the middle ear or mastoid may be treated with more aggressive surgery in the form a subtotal temporal bone resection (STBR), which extends the LTBR to include the ossicular chain, otic capsule, facial nerve, and all bone overlying the adjacent middle and posterior cranial fossa dura such that the stump of the internal auditory canal and bone of the petrous apex constitute the deep base of the surgical bed (**Fig. 2**). Although it is possible to achieve complete tumor resection via STBR, the nature of this procedure necessitates that it is undertaken at least in part by piecemeal dissection thereby clouding the status of surgical margins. Total or radical temporal bone resection involves further extension of STBR to include the carotid artery and jugular bulb-sigmoid, but this procedure is rarely indicated. Finally, each of these procedures may be given the prefix designation "extended" to include concurrent resection of additional adjacent structures such as the temporomandibular joint or styloid process.

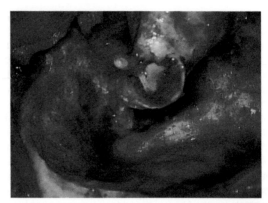

Fig. 1. Lateral temporal bone resection (*right ear*) involves en bloc resection of the bony and membranous external auditory canal, tympanic ring, tympanic membrane, and malleus ma-nubrium. If properly executed, the undersurface of the tympanic membrane should be intact as the specimen is rotated out of the surgical field and separated from the temporo-mandibular joint capsule.

Petrous apicectomy and infratemporal fossa exposure

In some instances, surgery requires extended anterior exposure into the petrous apex and infratemporal fossa beyond what is afforded by the standard temporal bone resection techniques.[9] Examples include cases that require mobilization of the intra-petrous carotid artery, tumors invading the pterygoid plates and musculature, and tu-mors with a significant inferior petrous apex component along the inferior petrosal sinus. In such instances, a lateral skull base approach to the infratemporal fossa is required (Fisch type B or C).[10] For malignant tumors, these approaches usually begin with blind sac closure of the ear canal with subtotal petrosectomy or with some form of

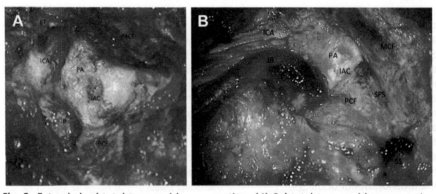

Fig. 2. Extended subtotal temporal bone resection. (*A*) Subtotal temporal bone resection (*left ear*) involves expansion of lateral temporal bone resection to include resection of the inner ear and facial nerve and removal of all bone off the middle cranial fossa (MCF) and posterior cranial fossa (PCF) dura. At the end of the resection, the petrous apex (PA), jugular bulb (JB), internal auditory canal (IAC), internal carotid artery (ICA), and membranous Eusta-chian tube (ET). The designation extended is given here because the resection also included removal of the mandibular condyle and drilling out of the glenoid fossa. (*B*) Subtotal tem-poral bone resection (*left ear*) can also be extended to include resection of the sigmoid sinus (SS) and jugular bulb if needed. SPS, superior petrosal sinus.

temporal bone resection as deemed necessary. The zygomatic arch is released via osteotomies (later reset with plates or permanently removed if a bulky free flap reconstruction is planned) so that the temporalis muscle can be reflected inferiorly. The glenoid fossa is exposed either by mandibular condylectomy or by disarticulation of the temporomandibular joint, yet the author's strong bias is to resect the condyle because the exposure afforded by disarticulation in children is limited by comparison and the long-term impact of condylectomy on mastication is not overwhelming. The soft tissue approach is finalized as the membranous Eustachian tube is transected.

Infratemporal fossa approaches allow the surgeon to perform a complete anterior petrosectomy progressing from lateral to medial without the need for brain retraction. After the glenoid fossa is drilled out, bone removal proceeds anterior and medial with sequential division of the middle meningeal artery and mandibular branch of the fifth cranial nerve. Last, broad access to the entire intrapetrous internal carotid artery is afforded up to foramen lacerum, as this is the chief advantage of this approach.[11] Dissection continues medially if dissection of the pterygoid plates and lateral nasopharyngeal wall is required (constituting transition from Fisch type B to a Fisch type C approach).[10,12]

Some malignant tumors isolated within the petrous apex may be approached in a way that preserves the ear canal and hearing mechanism. In these instances a preauricular approach to the infratemporal fossa (Fisch type D)[10] is possible, with the caveat that exposure afforded by this technique is considerably more narrow and that the child will have a lifetime requirement for a tympanostomy tube if the membranous Eustachian tube is violated. Alternatively, if tumor dissection does not require full carotid mobilization and the inferior petrous apex is uninvolved, a subtemporal approach (extended middle cranial fossa) can provide excellent exposure.[13] Although a subtemporal approach may require slight retraction of the temporal lobe, it avoids the significant morbidity associated with violation of the ear canal, otic capsule, temporomandibular joint, and mandibular branch of the fifth cranial nerve.[14]

Fisch partial mastoidotympanectomy

Some malignant tumors of the parotid and upper cervical lymph nodes that lie within the retromandibular fossa and poststyloid space can secondarily invade the inferior aspect of the temporal bone while sparing involvement of the external auditory canal. Such cases are ideal candidates for what has been described by Fisch and Mattox[10] as partial mastoidotympanectomy. This approach involves the sequence of intact canal wall mastoidectomy, decompression of the distal aspect of the mastoid segment of the facial nerve, amputation of the mastoid tip from the digastric muscle, and resection of the inferior tympanic bone and associated styloid base (**Fig. 3**). This final step includes elevation and preservation of the membranous external auditory canal followed by a drill out of the tympanic bone anterior to the facial nerve; this dissection extends just inferior to the tympanic ring and just lateral to the jugular bulb. Drilling of the styloid base augments medial exposure to the deep lobe of the parotid gland and the anterior aspect of the stylomastoid foramen. In doing so, the styloid process and muscular attachments are released for en bloc resection with the tumor specimen if desired. This approach greatly aids identification of the proximal extratemporal aspect of the facial nerve when bulky tumor is present and also provides a proximal margin for facial nerve grafting in cases in which tumor invasion necessitates nerve sacrifice. In the author's experience, it is critical to provide bulky inferior soft tissue support of the preserved membranous external auditory canal during the reconstructive phase in order to avoid postoperative canal breakdown and canal-mastoid fistula.

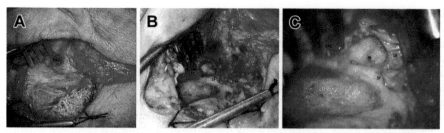

Fig. 3. Fisch partial mastoidotympanectomy. Parotid tumors of the retromandibular fossa and poststyloid space that invade the temporal bone from below while sparing the external auditory canal are ideal for this approach. (*A*) The mastoid and tympanic bone (*right side*) are exposed in continuum with the parotid fascia while preserving the membranous external auditory canal (EAC). Note that the parotid tumor is only minimally exposed at this point. (*B*) Intact canal wall mastoidectomy with skeletonization of the mastoid segment of the facial nerve and wide exposure of the stylomastoid foramen (SF) is undertaken. In doing so the mastoid tip is amputated from the digastric muscle (DM) and the tympanic bone is drilled anterior to the facial nerve until the jugular bulb (JB) is exposed inferior to the tympanic ring. Tympanic bone drilling will uncover the tumor (T). (*C*) This approach affords release the styloid process from styloid base (SB) and is also useful if facial nerve grafting is required.

Radiation Therapy

Radiation therapy is often a major component of pediatric temporal bone cancer treatment. Forms of external beam radiation, brachytherapy, and stereotactic radiosurgery have all been used within various treatment regimens, most often as part of a multimodality approach that may also include surgery, chemotherapy, or both. Of note, for most high-grade sarcomas that involve the temporal bone in children, especially RMSs, moderate to high doses of external beam radiation (5000–7000 cGy) are generally combined with multidrug chemotherapy after surgical resection. Radiation generally plays a postoperative adjuvant role at slightly lower doses in the treatment of surgically resectable temporal bone cancer, especially when margins are positive, disease is recurrent, regional lymph node metastasis is extensive, or aggressive histologic features are present.[15] Application of single-modality external beam radiation with curative intent would only rarely be considered for pediatric skull base cancers, usually certain lymphomas.

Negative effects of external beam radiation to the skull base in children can be considerable and may include impaired cranial bone growth, chronic headache, pituitary dysfunction, poor tooth development, cataracts, neurosensory hearing loss, Eustachian tube dysfunction, and osteoradionecrosis.[16] Whole brain exposure to external beam radiation in children may result in intellectual developmental impairment.[17] There is also an unspecified risk of developing a secondary radiation-induced benign tumor or malignancy later in life, especially in the thyroid gland.

Stereotactic radiosurgery, in its various forms, plays an adjuvant role in the treatment of skull base cancer.[18] Most often this has involved treatment of a low-grade tumor, such as a chordoma, that is located in a surgically inaccessible area, but there are also reports of stereotactic radiosurgery for high-grade tumor remnants within a previously radiated field. Indications for stereotactic radiosurgery in the temporal bone include residual or recurrent disease within the jugular foramen or perineural tumor spread into Meckel cave, the internal auditory canal, or the cavernous sinus.[18,19]

Chemotherapy

As with radiation therapy, multidrug chemotherapy often plays a vital role in the treatment of pediatric temporal bone cancer, especially sarcomas. In general, when surgical morbidity is deemed unacceptable, gross tumor resection is not feasible, or if distant metastases are present at the time of initial diagnosis, combined chemotherapy and radiation therapy are used as part of a primary nonsurgical treatment regimen. Particular chemotherapeutic regimens vary considerably depending on the underlying tumor pathology and disease extent, and discussion of the numerous chemotherapy drugs used to treat various forms of temporal bone malignancy is beyond the intended scope of this article. The toxicity and side effects of chemotherapy in children depend on the particular drugs in use, but mucositis, anemia, nausea, alopecia, and neutropenic fever are common.[20] Children receiving chemotherapy often require emotional and nutritional support, which specialized pediatric cancer centers may be particularly adept at providing.

CHARACTERISTICS OF SPECIFIC TEMPORAL BONE MALIGNANCIES
Rhabdomyosarcoma

RMS is a malignant tumor derived from embryologic skeletal muscle precursor cells that is almost exclusively seen in children. RMS is the most common type of pediatric temporal bone malignancy.[21] These tumors typically contain the proteins myoD1 and myogenin, both of which are found in embryologic skeletal muscle but not in the cells of developed skeletal muscle. RMS can occur in numerous locations, even where native skeletal muscle is not present. The head and neck region is a common site for RMS, accounting for roughly 35% to 40% of all RMSs, and the orbit is by far the most common site of origin within the head and neck (25%), followed by the paranasal sinuses and nasopharynx. By comparison, primary temporal bone RMSs account for less than 5% of RMSs that occur in the head and neck,[22] despite the fact that RMS is the by far the most common temporal bone malignancy in children.

Several descriptions of the histologic variants of RMS have been used over the years, but most modern depictions divide RMS into 3 main cellular classifications: embryonal rhabdomyosarcoma (ERMS), alveolar rhabdomyosarcoma (ARMS), and pleomorphic RMS (anaplastic).[23] Pleomorphic RMS is very rare and generally found in adults, not children, and therefore is not addressed further in this article. ERMS is further subdivided into spindle cell, botryoid, and embryonal (conventional) subtypes. From a practical standpoint, the most important subclass delineation with respect to clinical relevance is the differentiation between ERMS and ARMS because the prognosis for ERMS is much better. Among subtypes of ERMS, spindle cell and botryoid are less common than conventional embryonal tumors, and they portend a particularly favorable outlook. By far, conventional ERMS is the most common subtype found in the ear and temporal bone (**Fig. 4**).[1,24,25]

Based on the reported cases of temporal bone RMS, it seems that these tumors can originate from the middle ear, external auditory canal, or mastoid. There seems to be a tendency toward early involvement of the fallopian canal and subsequent intracranial extension by perineural spread through the internal auditory canal.[1] Direct extension into the cranial vault is also possible by tumor erosion of the tegmen tympani and tegmen mastoideum or by involvement of other cranial nerves in the jugular foramen or infratemporal fossa.[24]

The staging and classification of RMS is unique and somewhat complicated; however, it correlates well with risk and prognosis. The Soft Tissue Sarcoma Committee of

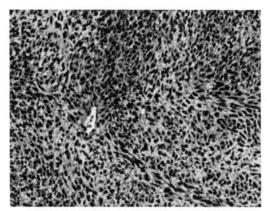

Fig. 4. Embryonal rhabdomyosarcoma. Hematoxylin-eosin stain of conventional rhabdo-myosarcoma demonstrating typical histologic features including sheets of small-spindled cells with eosinophilic cytoplasm and eccentric ovoid nuclei. Embryonal subtype rhabdo-myosarcoma is by far the most common variant encountered in the head and neck region (original magnification 10×).

the Children's Oncology Group (COG-STS) established the current staging process[26] that includes (1) assignment of an RMS tumor stage at the time of diagnosis based on clinical and radiologic features,[23,27] (2) assignment of an RMS group after surgery (if performed) based on completeness of resection and extent of any residual disease noted on histopathology,[28,29] (3) assignment of RMS risk classification determined by the RMS tumor stage, RMS group, and tumor histologic subtype.[30,31] The RMS risk classification in turn portrays prognosis and drives the aggressiveness of chemotherapy and radiation therapy.

Primary tumors are designated T1 unless they are invasive with extension beyond the site of origin into adjacent structures, in which case they are considered stage T2. Although data are not available for standardization of ear and temporal bone RMSs, tumors should probably be considered T2 if structures outside the external ear and tympanomastoid space are involved such as the mandible, dura, internal auditory canal, parotid, neck, or periauricular skin. Similarly, tumor extension through bone into the jugular foramen, petroclival junction, carotid canal, or occipital bone also seems worthy of upstage. Another "a" or "b" designation is given if the tumor is less than (T1a or T2a) or greater than (T1b or T2b) 5 cm in diameter. The primary tumor site of RMS is also designated as being favorable or unfavorable; temporal bone tumors are all by definition unfavorable (parameningeal) according to the COG-STS. Designations for regional lymph node metastasis and distant metastasis are N1 and M1, respectively, if either of these is present. With this information, RMS tumor stage is assigned according to **Table 2**.[23,27]

Stage	Site	T Stage	Size	Regional Lymph Nodes	Distant Metastasis
Table 2 **COG-STS: pretreatment RMS tumor stage**					
I	Favorable	T1 or T2	Any	N0 or N1	M0
II	Unfavorable	T1 or T2	a, ≤5 cm	N0	M0
III	Unfavorable	T1 or T2	a, ≤5 cm	N1	M0
			b, ≥5 cm	N0 or N1	
IV	Any	T1 or T2	Any	Any	M1

Ideally, RMS (irrespective of location) is treated by complete wide surgical resection with microscopically clear margins because the completeness of the resection determines RMS group assignment and in turn potentially affects RMS risk classification and prognosis. Because most temporal bone RMSs are not simply confined to the external auditory canal, en bloc resection via LTBR is usually not possible. Thus, extended LTBR or STBR with possible combined dissection into the infratemporal fossa is generally required if complete resection is attempted, involving at least some degree of piecemeal dissection as the drill passes through affected air cells with a requisite degree of margin ambiguity. Thus, in the author's opinion, even if separately sent surgical margins are tumor free, an honest assessment of tumor margins should render assignment of at least group II for most RMSs of the ear and temporal bone not solely confined to the external auditory canal according to **Table 3**.[28,29]

As depicted in **Table 4**, RMS tumor stage, RMS group, and tumor histology determine RMS risk assignment, which in turn determines prognosis.[30,31] The role of surgery for ear and temporal bone RMS is controversial because the morbidity associated with radical surgery may be quite significant and complete resection may be impossible.[32] Thus, surgery for temporal bone RMS may be limited to biopsy followed by primary chemoradiation at some treatment centers.[33] However, the author advocates attempted surgical resection in most cases if distant metastasis is absent. The rationale for this view is based on the fact that RMS risk classification for a typical tumor (RMS tumor stage II or III, embryonal histology, no distant metastasis) will be either low or intermediate, but which of these is assigned will hinge upon the nature of surgical resection. Even a gross total resection with microscopically positive margins (RMS group 2) renders an improved risk group assignment (low risk) as opposed to the situation (intermediate risk) in which no attempt is made at tumor resection (RMS group 3).

All children with RMS, even in the most favorable risk classification, receive some form of chemotherapy and most receive radiation therapy.[26] Owing to modern advances in the numerous drug regimens used to treat RMS, survival outcomes have seen marked improvement over the past few decades. For temporal bone RMS, whole brain radiation is avoided unless the brain itself is invaded, but medium to high radiation doses are given to the tumor bed and adjacent lymph node basins. The expected 5-year survival rate by RMS risk classification is as follows: low-risk group 90%, intermediate-risk group 60% to 80%, and high-risk group 20% to 40%.[31]

Table 3
COG-STS: surgical-pathologic RMS group system

Group	Definition
I	Localized tumor, completely removed with microscopically clear margins and no regional lymph node involvement
II	Localized tumor, completely removed with (1) microscopic disease at the margin; (2) regional disease with involved nodes, grossly removed regional lymph nodes without microresidual disease; or (3) regional disease with involved nodes, grossly removed but with microscopic residual and/or histologic involvement of the most distal node from the primary tumor
III	Localized tumor, incompletely removed with gross residual disease after (1) biopsy only or (2) gross major resection of the primary tumor (>50%)
IV	Distant metastases are present at diagnosis. This category includes (1) radiographically identified evidence of tumor spread and (2) positive tumor cells in cerebrospinal, pleural, or peritoneal fluids, or implants in these regions

Table 4 COG-STS: RMS risk classification			
Risk	**Histology**	**Tumor Stage**	**Group**
Low risk	Embryonal	I	I, II, III
		II, III	I, II
Intermediate risk	Embryonal	II, III	III
	Alveolar	I, II, III	I, II, III
High risk	Any	IV	IV

Other Sarcomas

Nonrhabdomyosarcomatous sarcoma (NRMSS) is extremely rare in the ear and temporal bone.[25] NRMSS accounts for only 7% of all head and neck malignancies in children, with a mere 10% of these having a skull base component.[21] Some of the NRMSSs that have been reported to occur in the ear and temporal bone of children and adolescents include chondrosarcoma,[34,35] chordoma,[36] osteosarcoma,[37,38] Ewing sarcoma,[39] fibrosarcoma, angiosarcoma, and chloroma (granulocytic sarcoma)[40]; however, determination of the mesenchymal cell of origin is not always possible.[21] Most sarcomas have high- and low-grade histologic variants, which affect the disease presentation and survival outlook. In contrast to RMS, low-grade NRMSSs are generally diagnosed as slow-growing lesions having an insidious onset of symptoms such as headache, otalgia, tinnitus, and cranial neuropathy. In particular, involvement of the sixth cranial nerve with associated diplopia on lateral gaze or involvement of the mandibular branch of the fifth cranial nerve with associated numbness along the lower part of the face and mandible is typical for chondrosarcoma or other NRMSSs involving the petrous apex. Past radiation therapy seems to be a risk factor for developing a sarcoma; Paget disease is a particular risk factor for cranial osteosarcoma.[41] Treatment of NRMSS is less controversial than that of RMS. Although it varies depending on the subtype and extent of disease, as a general rule, wide surgical excision followed by postoperative chemotherapy and/or radiation therapy is favored.[21] However, all these tumors are extraordinarily rare; thus, well-defined treatment protocols for those with ear and skull base involvement do not exist.

Among NRMSSs, chordoma merits some particular discussion.[36] Although there is some minor controversy regarding the proper classification of chordoma, most agree that it is properly considered to be a sarcoma derived from remnants of the embryologic notochord.[42] These tumors come in 3 different histologic subtypes (classical, chondroid, and dedifferentiated), which along with location defines their classification. In the skull base, an overwhelming majority of chordomas arise from the clivus and are generally considered tumors of the anterior skull base. However, secondary involvement of the petroclival junction and temporal bone may occur, as do rare variants arise primarily from within the lateral part of the skull base. Chordomas tend to be deeply infiltrative and difficult to definitively resect, but are usually low grade and slow growing. In children, the prognosis in those younger than 5 years seems to differ markedly from that in older children because infants have a higher rate of metastasis (60% vs 9%) and worse survival outlook.[36]

Lymphoma and Carcinoma

Although rare in the temporal bone, lymphoma is the most common type of head and neck cancer encountered in children, and overall, lymphoma accounts for 10% to 15% of all childhood malignancies.[43] Most of these (60%) are non-Hodgkin lymphoma.[44] Imaging is useful in these cases to help differentiate lymphoma from sarcoma or carcinoma with findings of homogeneous tumor that are isointense to brain on T2 MRI images and highly attenuating with smooth borders on CT being typical.[45] For most cases of lymphoma that involve the temporal bone, there is also disease involvement at another site within the head and neck—often a site more easily approached for a biopsy. As with most lymphomas in the head and neck, surgery is limited to tissue biopsy to establish a diagnosis and to prompt primary chemotherapy and/or radiation therapy.

Carcinomas of the temporal bone are incredibly rare in children. If present, these tumors generally arise from the skin of the ear canal, cutaneous appendages, or middle ear mucosa. Basal cell carcinoma can also occur as part of nevoid basal cell carcinoma syndrome, also known as Gorlin-Goltz syndrome.[46] Unlike sarcomas, which may originate from structures deep within the skull base, carcinomas tend to occur in areas where they may become symptomatic at an earlier stage. Thus, the feasibility of complete surgical resection of carcinoma is often more favorable than that of sarcoma. The outlook for early-stage squamous cell carcinoma confined to the external auditory canal is quite favorable with aggressive treatment, which typically involves LTBR with or without postoperative radiation therapy. For reference, 5-year survival in adults with early-stage squamous cell carcinoma of the ear canal ranges from 80% to 100%.[47] However, survival drops significantly if there is tumor extension outside the external auditory canal, regional lymph node involvement, local disease recurrence, or distant metastasis.

Parotid Tumors with Secondary Temporal Bone Invasion

Parotid cancer in children has an annual incidence of 1.43 cases per million. Most affected children are older than 10 years. Overwhelmingly, the 2 most common tumor subtypes are mucoepidermoid carcinoma (49%) and acinic cell carcinoma (40%)[48]; however, RMS of the parotid also exists (**Fig. 5**). As is the case with adults, large

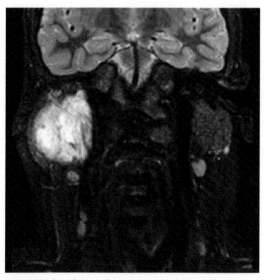

Fig. 5. Rhabdomyosarcoma involving the temporal bone. Short tau inversion recovery sequence coronal MRI image of right-sided rhabdomyosarcoma involving the temporal bone and parotid gland.

parotid tumors can invade the ear secondarily such that otic signs and symptoms may be the presenting manifestations. Treatment of malignant parotid tumors that invade the ear and temporal bone usually consists of temporal bone resection in addition to some form of parotidectomy followed by postoperative radiation therapy.[15] Parotid tumors of the retromandibular fossa and poststyloid space that spare the external auditory canal may benefit from Fisch partial mastoidotympanectomy in lieu of LTBR in order to preserve hearing while providing improved tumor exposure. Long-term survival of children affected by malignant parotid tumors is generally favorable.[48]

SUMMARY

Ear and temporal bone cancer presents a unique challenge in children because of its rarity. RMS is the most common temporal bone malignancy encountered in the pediatric population, the assessment of which is a standardized process that considers tumor location, surgical-pathologic assessment, and histologic subtype. The treatment of choice for most localized malignant tumors of the ear and temporal bone is wide surgical resection followed by chemotherapy and radiation therapy; however, the decision to perform radical surgery must take into account surgical risk, prognosis, and associated morbidity.

REFERENCES

1. Sbeity S, Abella A, Arcand P, et al. Temporal bone rhabdomyosarcoma in children. Int J Pediatr Otorhinolaryngol 2007;71:807–14.
2. Gidley PW, Thompson CR, Roberts DB, et al. The oncology of otology. Laryngoscope 2012;122:393–400.
3. Irving RM, Broadbent V, Jones NS. Langerhans' cell histiocytosis in childhood: management of head and neck manifestations. Laryngoscope 1994;104:64–70.
4. Donadieu J, Chalard F, Jeziorski E. Medical management of Langerhans cell histiocytosis from diagnosis to treatment. Expert Opin Pharmacother 2012;13: 1309–22.
5. Gil Z, Constantini S, Spektor S, et al. Skull base approaches in the pediatric population. Head Neck 2005;27:682–9.
6. Eppley BL, Morales L, Wood R, et al. Resorbable PLLA-PGA plate and screw fixation in pediatric craniofacial surgery: clinical experience in 1883 patients. Plast Reconstr Surg 2004;114:850–6 [discussion: 857].
7. Gharb BB, Salgado CJ, Moran SL, et al. Free anterolateral thigh flap in pediatric patients. Ann Plast Surg 2011;66:143–7.
8. Metrailer AM, Gluth MB. Lateral temporal bone resection. In: Kountakis SE, editor. Encyclopedia of otolaryngology, head & neck surgery. New York (NY): Springer; 2013. p. 1458–62.
9. Gluth MB, Kutz JW. Petrous apicectomy. In: Kountakis SE, editor. Encyclopedia of otolaryngology, head & neck surgery. New York (NY): Springer; 2013. p. 2134–42.
10. Fisch U, Mattox D. Microsurgery of the skull base. New York: Thieme; 1988.
11. Fisch U. Infratemporal fossa approach to tumours of the temporal bone and base of the skull. J Laryngol Otol 1978;92:949–67.
12. Fisch U. The infratemporal fossa approach for nasopharyngeal tumors. Laryngoscope 1983;93:36–44.
13. Sekhar LN, Schramm VL Jr, Jones NF. Subtemporal-preauricular infratemporal fossa approach to large lateral and posterior cranial base neoplasms. J Neurosurg 1987;67:488–99.

14. Leonetti JP, Anderson DE, Marzo SJ, et al. The preauricular subtemporal approach for transcranial petrous apex tumors. Otol Neurotol 2008;29:380–3.
15. Gidley PW, DeMonte F. Temporal bone malignancies. Neurosurg Clin N Am 2013; 24:97–110.
16. Larson DL, Kroll S, Jaffe N, et al. Long-term effects of radiotherapy in childhood and adolescence. Am J Surg 1990;160:348–51.
17. Silber JH, Radcliffe J, Peckham V, et al. Whole-brain irradiation and decline in intelligence: the influence of dose and age on IQ score. J Clin Oncol 1992;10: 1390–6.
18. Miller RC, Foote RL, Coffey RJ, et al. The role of stereotactic radiosurgery in the treatment of malignant skull base tumors. Int J Radiat Oncol Biol Phys 1997;39: 977–81.
19. Krishnan S, Foote RL, Brown PD, et al. Radiosurgery for cranial base chordomas and chondrosarcomas. Neurosurgery 2005;56:777–84 [discussion: 777–84].
20. LeBaron S, Zeltzer LK, LeBaron C, et al. Chemotherapy side effects in pediatric oncology patients: drugs, age, and sex as risk factors. Med Pediatr Oncol 1988; 16:263–8.
21. Lyos AT, Goepfert H, Luna MA, et al. Soft tissue sarcoma of the head and neck in children and adolescents. Cancer 1996;77:193–200.
22. Turner JH, Richmon JD. Head and neck rhabdomyosarcoma: a critical analysis of population-based incidence and survival data. Otolaryngol Head Neck Surg 2011;145:967–73.
23. Lawrence W Jr, Anderson JR, Gehan EA, et al. Pretreatment TNM staging of childhood rhabdomyosarcoma: a report of the Intergroup Rhabdomyosarcoma Study Group. Children's Cancer Study Group. Pediatric Oncology Group. Cancer 1997;80:1165–70.
24. Wiatrak BJ, Pensak ML. Rhabdomyosarcoma of the ear and temporal bone. Laryngoscope 1989;99:1188–92.
25. Naufal PM. Primary sarcomas of the temporal bone. Arch Otolaryngol 1973;98: 44–50.
26. Malempati S, Hawkins DS. Rhabdomyosarcoma: review of the Children's Oncology Group (COG) Soft-Tissue Sarcoma Committee experience and rationale for current COG studies. Pediatr Blood Cancer 2012;59:5–10.
27. Lawrence W Jr, Gehan EA, Hays DM, et al. Prognostic significance of staging factors of the UICC staging system in childhood rhabdomyosarcoma: a report from the Intergroup Rhabdomyosarcoma Study (IRS-II). J Clin Oncol 1987;5: 46–54.
28. Crist WM, Garnsey L, Beltangady MS, et al. Prognosis in children with rhabdomyosarcoma: a report of the intergroup rhabdomyosarcoma studies I and II. Intergroup Rhabdomyosarcoma Committee. J Clin Oncol 1990;8:443–52.
29. Crist W, Gehan EA, Ragab AH, et al. The third intergroup rhabdomyosarcoma study. J Clin Oncol 1995;13:610–30.
30. Raney RB, Anderson JR, Barr FG, et al. Rhabdomyosarcoma and undifferentiated sarcoma in the first two decades of life: a selective review of intergroup rhabdomyosarcoma study group experience and rationale for Intergroup Rhabdomyosarcoma Study V. J Pediatr Hematol Oncol 2001;23:215–20.
31. Breneman JC, Lyden E, Pappo AS, et al. Prognostic factors and clinical outcomes in children and adolescents with metastatic rhabdomyosarcoma–a report from the Intergroup Rhabdomyosarcoma Study IV. J Clin Oncol 2003;21:78–84.
32. Goepfert H, Cangir A, Lindberg R, et al. Rhabdomyosarcoma of the temporal bone. Is surgical resection necessary? Arch Otolaryngol 1979;105:310–3.

33. Durve DV, Kanegaonkar RG, Albert D, et al. Paediatric rhabdomyosarcoma of the ear and temporal bone. Clin Otolaryngol Allied Sci 2004;29:32–7.

34. Koch BB, Karnell LH, Hoffman HT, et al. National cancer database report on chondrosarcoma of the head and neck. Head Neck 2000;22:408–25.

35. Gadwal SR, Fanburg-Smith JC, Gannon FH, et al. Primary chondrosarcoma of the head and neck in pediatric patients: a clinicopathologic study of 14 cases with a review of the literature. Cancer 2000;88:2181–8.

36. Borba LA, Al-Mefty O, Mrak RE, et al. Cranial chordomas in children and adolescents. J Neurosurg 1996;84:584–91.

37. Price CH, Jeffree GM. Incidence of bone sarcoma in SW England, 1946-74, in relation to age, sex, tumour site and histology. Br J Cancer 1977;36:511–22.

38. Sharma SC, Handa KK, Panda N, et al. Osteogenic sarcoma of the temporal bone. Am J Otolaryngol 1997;18:220–3.

39. Watanabe H, Tsubokawa T, Katayama Y, et al. Primary Ewing's sarcoma of the temporal bone. Surg Neurol 1992;37:54–8.

40. Levy R, Shvero J, Sandbank J. Granulocytic sarcoma (chloroma) of the temporal bone. Int J Pediatr Otorhinolaryngol 1989;18:163–9.

41. Thompson JB, Patterson RH Jr, Parsons H. Sarcomas of the calvaria; surgical experience with 14 patients. J Neurosurg 1970;32:534–8.

42. Wold LE, Laws ER Jr. Cranial chordomas in children and young adults. J Neurosurg 1983;59:1043–7.

43. Sandlund JT, Downing JR, Crist WM. Non-Hodgkin's lymphoma in childhood. N Engl J Med 1996;334:1238–48.

44. Young JL Jr, Ries LG, Silverberg E, et al. Cancer incidence, survival, and mortality for children younger than age 15 years. Cancer 1986;58:598–602.

45. Choi HK, Cheon JE, Kim IO, et al. Central skull base lymphoma in children: MR and CT features. Pediatr Radiol 2008;38:863–7.

46. Gorlin RJ. Nevoid basal cell carcinoma syndrome. Dermatol Clin 1995;13:113–25.

47. Gidley PW, Roberts DB, Sturgis EM. Squamous cell carcinoma of the temporal bone. Laryngoscope 2010;120:1144–51.

48. Allan BJ, Tashiro J, Diaz S, et al. Malignant tumors of the parotid gland in children: incidence and outcomes. J Craniofac Surg 2013;24:1660–4.

Index

Note: Page numbers of article titles are in **boldface** type.

A

Adenoma, middle ear, 305–306
Adenomatous tumors, of middle ear, biologic behavior of, 306
    classification of, 310–311
    clinical presentation of, 306–307
    diagnosis of, 307
    imaging of, 307–308
    microscopy and immunohistochemistry of, 309–310
    outcome/prognosis of, 312–313
    pathogenesis of, 308–309
    treatment of, 311–312
Arterial spin labeling, for diagnosis of arteriovenous fistulas and arteriovenous
    malformations, 274–276
Arteriovenous fistulas, and arteriovenous malformations, arterial spin labeling
    for diagnosis of, 274–276
Arteriovenous malformations, and arteriovenous fistulas, arterial spin labeling
    for diagnosis of, 274–276

B

Bone malignancies, pediatric temporal, characteristics of, 383–388
    chemotherapy in, 383
    ear and, 376–377
    evaluation and diagnosis of, 377, 378
    microsurgery in, 377–381, 382
        Fisch partial mastoidotympanectomy for, 381, 382
        petrous apicectomy and infratemporal fossa exposure for, 380–381
        temporal bone resection for, 379, 380
    presentation of, 376–377
    radiation therapy in, 382
    rhabdomyosarcoma and, **375–390**
    treatment of, 377–383

C

Carcinoma, of head and neck, in children, 386–387
Cholesteatoma, complications of, 270
    evaluation of, high-resolution computed tomography for, 264–266
        imaging techniques for, 264–266
        magnetic resonance imaging for, 266–267
    imaging of, indications for, 268–270
    postoperative surveillance of, 269–270

Otolaryngol Clin N Am 48 (2015) 391–395
http://dx.doi.org/10.1016/S0030-6665(15)00011-0
0030-6665/15/$ – see front matter © 2015 Elsevier Inc. All rights reserved.

oto.theclinics.com

Cholesteatoma (*continued*)
    preoperative assessment of, 268–269
Cholesterol granuloma, and petrous apex lesions, **361–373**
Chondrosarcomas, 344, 349, 355
Chordomas, 344, 349, 355
Collet-Sicard syndrome, 345
Computed tomography, high-resolution, for evaluation of cholesteatoma
    and epidermoids, 264–266

E

Ear, and pediatric temporal bone malignancy, 376–377
    middle, adenomatous tumors of. See *Adenomatous tumors, of middle ear.*
Endolymphatic sac tumors, **317–330**, 344, 346, 349, 356
    and other inner ear tumors, clinical distinction between, 318, 319
    clinical presentation of, 318–320
    grading and treatment system for, 323
    histology of, 322–323
    imaging of, 320, 321–322
    in Von Hippel-Lindau disease, 322
    staging of, 323–324
    surgical management of, institutional experiences with, 327
    treatment of, 324–327
Epidermoids, evaluation of, high-resolution computed tomography for, 264–266
        imaging techniques for, 264–266
        magnetic resonance imaging for, 266–267
    imaging of, indications for, 268–270

G

Glomus tympanicum tumors, **293–304**
    additional workup in, 299
    demographics and clinical evaluation of, 297
    diagnostic imaging and staging of, 297–298, 299, 300
    histology and pathophysiology of, 295–296
    history of, 294–295
    of head and neck, 294
    of middle ear, 293
    prognosis in, 301
    surgical resection of, 294
    treatment of, 299–301

H

Head and neck, lymphoma and carcinoma of, in children, 386–387

J

Jugular foramen, paragangliomas of. See *Paraganglioma(s), of jugular foramen.*
Jugular foramen tumors, nonparaganglioma, **343–359**
        epidemiology of, 343

    evaluation and diagnosis of, 346–347
    imaging characteristics of, 347–350, 351
    microsurgery in, 350–353
        infratemporal fossa approach for, 352
        retrosigmoid craniotomy for, 352–353
        transcochlear approach for, 352–353
        translabyrinthine approach for, 352
    observation in, 354–355
    outcomes of, cranial neuropathy, 356
        recurrence, 356
    presentation of, 345–346
    radiotherapy in, 353–354
    treatment of, 350–355

L

Lymphoma, of head and neck, in children, 386–387

M

Magnetic resonance imaging, for evaluation of cholesteatoma and
    epidermoids, 266–267
Meningiomas, jugular foramen, 344, 345, 355

N

Neurotologists, communication with patients, Breen on, 258–259
        Vrabec on, 259
    critical analysis of, Breen on, 261
        Vrabec on, 261
    efficiency of, Breen on, 260
        Vrabec on, 260–261
    judgment of, Breen on, 259
        Vrabec on, 259–260
    lifetime learning by, Breen on, 262
        Vrabec on, 262
    responsibility of, Breen on, 258
        Vrabec on, 258
Neurotology, early practice of, **257–262**

P

Paraganglioma(s), imaging of, novel radiotracers of, 273–274
    jugular, contemporary management of, **331–341**
        disease presentaion of, 332, 333
        genetic screening in, 333–334
        imaging of, 333, 334, 335, 336
        management of, embolization in, 335–336, 337
            observation in, 338
            radiation in, 337–338
            surgery in, 336–337

Paraganglioma(s) (*continued*)
    Otology Group of Vanderbilt experience with, 338–339
        observation in, 339
        radiation in, 339
        surgery and, 338
    tumor classification of, 333
    of jugular foramen, angiography and embolization of, 271–272
        high-resolution computed tomography of, 270–271
        magnetic resonance imaging of, 271
        nuclear medicine imaging of, 272–273
        whole-body molecular imaging of, 270–273
    tympanic. See *Glomus tympanicum tumors.*
Parotid tumors, with secondary temporal bone invasion, 387–388
Petrous apex lesions, cholesterol granuloma and, **361–373**
    computed tomography of, 363, 366
    diagnosis and management of, 361–362
    epidemiology and pathophysiology of, 362
    evaluation and diagnosis of, 362–363
    magnetic resonance imaging of, 363–367
    management of, 367–368
        extradural middle fossa approach to, 368
        hearing preservation transtemporal approaches to, 368–370
        nonhearing transtemporal approaches to, 370
        transnasal endoscopic approach to, 370
    outcomes and prognosis in, 370–371
    presentation of, 362–363
    radiographic studies in, 363, 364–365

    R

Radiotracers, novel, for imaging of paragangliomas, 273–274
Rhabdomyosarcoma, and other pediatric temporal bone malignancies, **375–390**
    characteristics of, 383–386
    classification of, 383
    involving temporal bone, 387–388
    primary, 384
    risk classification, 385, 386
    treatment of, 385

    S

Sarcoma, nonrhabdomyosarcomatous, 386
Schwannomas, jugular foramen, 344, 345, 348–349, 355
Skull base tumors, management of, 257
Squamous cell carcinoma, of temporal bone. See *Temporal bone, squamous cell carcinoma of.*

    T

Temporal bone, secondary invasion of, parotid tumors with, 387–388
    squamous cell carcinoma of, **281–292**

    adjuvant therapies in, 289–290
    case history of, 281–284, 285, 286
    diagnosis of, 285–287
        biopsy in, 284, 286
        imaging in, 285–286
        metastatic workup in, 286–287
    en bloc versus piecemeal removal of, 288–289
    facial nerve management in, 290
    palliative therapy in, indications for, 290
    parotidectomy and neck dissection in, 289
    presentation of, 284, 286
    prognosis in, 290–291
    staging of, 287
    surgical margins in, importance of, 290
    treatment of, 287–291
Temporal bone disorders, imaging innovations in, **263–280**

V

Vernet syndrome, 345
Villaret syndrome, 345
Von Hippel-Lindau disease, 320–322

Moving?

Make sure your subscription moves with you!

To notify us of your new address, find your **Clinics Account Number** (located on your mailing label above your name), and contact customer service at:

Email: journalscustomerservice-usa@elsevier.com

800-654-2452 (subscribers in the U.S. & Canada)
314-447-8871 (subscribers outside of the U.S. & Canada)

Fax number: 314-447-8029

Elsevier Health Sciences Division
Subscription Customer Service
3251 Riverport Lane
Maryland Heights, MO 63043

*To ensure uninterrupted delivery of your subscription, please notify us at least 4 weeks in advance of move.

Printed and bound by CPI Group (UK) Ltd, Croydon, CR0 4YY

07/10/2024

01040498-0014